The Kidney Disease Solution

Achieve optimal kidney health with these simple steps

By

Dr. Abdy Fari

•Conclusion

Introduction

Your kidneys are very important organs that do a lot of important things in your body. They filter waste and fluids from your blood, control your blood pressure, make hormones, and keep your body's electrolytes in balance. It is essential for your overall health and well-being to maintain healthy kidneys; however, kidney disease is unfortunately becoming more prevalent worldwide, affecting millions of people annually.

The kidneys' primary function is to cleanse the blood and return it to the body with clean blood. Every moment around one liter of blood - one-fifth of all the blood siphoned by the heart - enters the kidneys through the renal veins. The renal veins are where the blood returns to the body after it has been cleaned.

About one million tiny nephrons are found in each kidney. A very small filter known as a glomerulus is attached to a tubule in each nephron. As blood goes through the nephron, liquid and byproducts are sifted through. A significant part of the liquid is then gotten back to the blood, while the side-effects are moved in any additional liquid as pee (small).

The ureter is a tube through which the urine enters the bladder. Through a tube called the urethra, urine exits the body from the bladder. The kidney ordinarily makes one to two liters of pee constantly contingent upon your fabricate, the amount you drink, the temperature and how much activity you do.

The work capacity of a healthy kidney can be significantly increased. Each kidney performs 50% of normal kidney function when there are two healthy kidneys. In the event that one kidney is lost, the other kidney can broaden and give up to 75 percent of the typical kidney capability (crafted by one and a half regularly working kidneys).

Luckily, there are straightforward advances you can take to accomplish ideal kidney wellbeing and decrease your gamble of creating kidney sickness. We'll take a look at these steps in this guide and give you the information you need to keep your kidneys healthy. These actions, which are simple to incorporate into your daily routine and can have a significant impact on your kidney health, range from drinking enough water and eating a well-balanced diet to regularly exercising and learning to manage stress.

You might be one of numerous to have been as of late determined to have kidney stones. You are in good company: You do not have to accept poor health because you have the ability to alter your lifestyle; many others are in the same situation. Kidney problems do have painful side effects. But the solutions are the same. Don't give up on living with kidney disease. Taking care of your kidney issues now can help you avoid problems in the future.

Kidney illness is a typical issue influencing around 10% of the total populace. The kidneys are powerful, small, bean-shaped organs that carry out numerous essential functions. They are in charge of a lot of important things, like filtering out waste, releasing hormones that control blood pressure, keeping the body's fluids in balance, and making urine. These vital organs can become damaged in a variety of ways. Kidney disease is most commonly caused by diabetes and high blood pressure. However, other risk factors include obesity, smoking, gender, age, and genetics. Uncontrolled glucose and hypertension harm veins in the kidneys, lessening their capacity to ideally work.

This guide is for you whether you have already been diagnosed with kidney disease or just want to take preventative measures. You can improve your kidney function, lower your risk of complications, and have better overall health and wellbeing by following these straightforward steps. Let's get started, then!

Understanding the significance of kidney health is essential for sustaining overall health. On either side of the spine, just below the ribcage, are the two tiny kidneys. They are essential for regulating blood pressure, balancing electrolytes, and removing waste and excess fluid from the body. Additionally, the kidneys produce hormones that control blood pressure, promote bone health, and regulate the production of red blood cells.

At the point when the kidneys are not working as expected, poisons and waste items collect in the blood, prompting a scope of medical issues. High blood pressure, diabetes, infections, autoimmune disorders, genetic predisposition, and kidney disease are all potential causes.

Kidney disease can be slowed down and prevented from progressing to heart disease, stroke, and kidney failure if it is detected and treated early. As a result, adopting healthy lifestyle habits like drinking enough water, eating a well-balanced diet, exercising frequently, controlling blood pressure, quitting smoking and drinking less alcohol, getting enough sleep, managing stress, and regularly monitoring kidney health are essential for maintaining kidney health.

The kidneys' primary function is to eliminate waste products and excess fluid from the body, as most people are aware. The urine removes these waste products and excess fluid. The excretion and reabsorption processes that lead to the production of urine are extremely intricate. The body's chemical balance must remain stable through this process.

The kidneys control the body's salt, potassium, and acid levels, which is crucial. Hormones that affect how other organs work are also made by the kidneys. For instance, red blood cell production is stimulated by a hormone produced by the kidneys. The kidneys also make other hormones that help regulate calcium metabolism and control blood pressure.

The vast majority won't see in the event that their kidneys are working somewhat less well than they used to in light of the fact that this doesn't as a rule cause side effects or prevent the kidneys from working. The majority of people's kidney function is affected only slightly and stays stable for many years. Only a small number of people's kidney function quickly deteriorates and will cause health issues. According to a May 2017 report from the British Kidney Patients Association, approximately one in eight people in the UK have some degree of kidney impairment—that is, their kidneys are not functioning as well as they once did. For the majority of these people, this will never be a major issue. This mild kidney impairment can worsen in some people, necessitating treatment for their kidneys. All kidney weakness, whether it be gentle or serious, is these days alluded to by specialists as 'ongoing kidney infection'.

There are numerous issues with the term "chronic kidney disease," which is frequently abbreviated as "CKD." Although in medical terminology the term "chronic" refers to a condition that lasts for a long time rather than something that can be treated quickly (an "acute" condition), many people interpret the term "chronic" to mean severe. Patients may experience unnecessary anxiety as a result of this misunderstanding, as they may believe their kidney function is worse than it actually is. Additionally, some medical professionals contend that impaired kidney function is not itself a disease. Instead, it's a sign that a person may be more likely to have other health issues, in the same way that high cholesterol levels aren't a disease in and of themselves but do raise the risk of cardiovascular disease.

chapter 1

Stay hydrated

Drinking enough water and other fluids to keep hydrated is essential to avoid dehydration. Your age, gender, weight, level of activity, and climate all influence how much water you need. Adults should drink at least 8 glasses (or 64 ounces) of water each day, but this amount can vary depending on individual requirements.

You may have been advised to consume eight glasses of water per day. That advice is reasonable, but it doesn't take into account every person's needs, like how active they are, their environment, and other things.

Up to 60% of our bodies are made of water. We lose water continually through our skin, pee, waste and sweat - in any event, when we relax. Water consumption has many advantages, including:

Maintaining a healthy internal body temperature, metabolizing food, regulating hunger, lubricating joints,

flushing bodily waste, and producing sufficient saliva
are all functions of saliva. If you don't drink enough
water, you run the risk of becoming dehydrated, which
can result in problems like impaired kidney function and
unbalanced electrolytes.

How much water should an individual consume daily?

Food accounts for approximately 20% of our daily fluid
intake, while beverages account for the remaining
portion.

How much water admission you want relies upon the sex
you were relegated upon entering the world. The U.S.
National Academies of Science, Engineering, and
Medicine recommend that men consume 3.7 liters
(roughly 16 cups) of fluid each day, while women
should consume 2.7 liters (roughly 11 cups). If you
sweat, exercise, or have a fever, diarrhea, or vomiting,
you need to drink even more water.

It is possible to drink too much water, although this is
uncommon. Especially for those with heart disease or
electrolyte abnormalities, an excess of water can be fatal.

The best course of action is to discuss with your doctor the optimal water intake for your body and activity level.

Tips for staying hydrated

1.In the morning, drink a glass of water. This gets your digestion running and gives you a jolt of energy. If you struggle with nighttime urination or heartburn, don't drink water before bed.

2.Buy a fancy or fun water bottle. A good water bottle can help you remember to drink more water throughout the day by showing you. As water levels drop, some bottles have words of encouragement printed on the side or marked measurements for monitoring intake.

3.Make use of notifications or alarms to your advantage. Throughout the day, use your smart devices to set alarms or notifications as reminders. Set your Google or Alexa device to remind you and give you verbal, encouraging words for a mental boost.

4.Center around your body's signs. Pay attention to whether your body is hungry or thirsty. Because we mistake thirst for hunger, we occasionally overeat.

5.Drink a glass of water before every feast. It will assist you in maintaining adequate hydration, improve food digestion, and speed up the feeling of fullness.

6.Add a flavor without calories. To make your water more appealing, try infusing it with fruits or vegetables. To make it easier to fill your water bottle in the morning, prepare a jug to infuse overnight in the refrigerator. For flavor on the go, pick up a water bottle with an integrated infusion basket.

7.Examine the hue of your urine. Throughout the day, some people check to see if their urine is clear or light in color. For some, dark yellow urine may indicate dehydration.

8.Trade high sugar drinks for shining water or seltzer. You will not only cut back on sugar that isn't necessary, but you will also drink more water.

9.Set a daily objective. You can stay motivated and work toward sustaining a healthy habit by setting a simple daily goal.

10.Make it difficult. Invite your friends to participate in a healthy competition to see who consistently achieves their daily goals.

10 Reasons Why Hydration is Important

Staying hydrated is an essential, yet frequently neglected, aspect of health maintenance. It becomes even more significant with age. There are a number of factors that increase the likelihood of dehydration in adults over the age of 60, including changes in body composition and natural drops in thirst. Diuretics and other drugs that make the body lose fluids are also more common in older people.

On the off chance that you're attempting to get eight 8-ounce glasses of water a day — the sum suggested by numerous wellbeing specialists — the following are 10 smart motivations to drink more.

1. Improved brain performance Memory, mood, concentration, and reaction time can all be affected by even mild dehydration—as little as 2% fluid loss. Even if you only drink a few glasses of water every day, it can help you think clearly, keep your emotions in check, and even fight anxiety. This is especially important for elderly people, who are more likely to become dehydrated and have trouble thinking straight.

2. Stomach related amicability
Your body needs water to appropriately process food. Without enough, you might encounter unpredictable solid discharges, gas, bulging, indigestion, and different inconveniences that can hurt your personal satisfaction. Increasing your liquid admission might assist with getting things going in the correct heading once more. It maintains proper digestion by assisting in the breakdown of dietary soluble fiber. Mineral water is especially beneficial; look for sodium and magnesium-enriched products.

3. More energy Dehydration can hinder oxygen delivery to the brain and slow down circulation. Your heart may also have to work harder to distribute oxygen throughout

your body if you don't drink enough fluids. All of that exhausted energy can cause you to feel drained, languid, and less engaged. You can avoid dehydration and have more energy to get you through the day by simply drinking more water.

4. Weight loss and management because it makes you feel full, drinking water between meals can keep you from reaching for the snack drawer. Your metabolism may also benefit from it. Drinking more water before each meal led to significant weight, body mass index, and body composition reductions in overweight women, according to one study. Another study from 2016 found that adults who increased their water intake by just one percent ate fewer calories. They also consumed less sugar, cholesterol, sodium, and saturated fat overall.

5. Reduced joint pain Did you know that approximately 80 percent of the cartilage in our joints is water? Your joints will stay well-lubricated if you drink enough water to keep them hydrated. This helps reduce friction by creating more of a "cushion" between the bones. Less contact implies smoother-moving joints and less a throbbing painfulness.

6. Better temperature regulation The body stores more heat when it is dehydrated, according to research. As a result, your tolerance for high temperatures decreases. When you're overheating during an activity, drinking a lot of water helps you sweat, which helps your body cool down. This implicit cooling component is basic in forestalling heat stroke and other possibly lethal intensity related conditions.

7. Kidney stone avoidance
Kidney stones are clusters of mineral gems that structure in the urinary lot. Assuming that you've at any point experienced one, you know how difficult they can be. Drinking enough water every day can help reduce the likelihood of developing stones by diluting the concentration of minerals in your urinary tract. Additionally, drinking water can assist in the prevention of urinary tract infections (UTIs) by flushing out harmful bacteria from your bladder.

8. Better heart health Your blood is mostly water, and if you don't drink enough of it, it gets concentrated, which can make an imbalance of important minerals

(electrolytes) in your body. Potassium and sodium, two of these minerals, are essential to the health of your heart.

9. Better detoxification Drinking a lot of water helps your body's natural detoxification processes, which help get rid of waste and harmful substances through urination, breathing, sweating, and bowel movements. Boosting your overall health by assisting your own potent internal detoxification processes can be beneficial.

10. Fewer headaches In some people, even a small amount of fluid loss can cause the brain to contract away from the skull, resulting in headaches and migraines. Drinking plenty of water on a regular basis may help alleviate headaches.

Food varieties that hydrate you

Your body regularly gets around 20% of the water it needs from the food sources you eat over the course of the day. Raw vegetables and fruits typically have the highest water content of any food. A diet high in produce is a good way to get more vitamins, minerals, and fiber into your body while also drinking more water every day.

A great choice are any fruits and vegetables that contain more than 80% water. However, when it comes to getting the amount of water your body needs, these foods all of which contain more than 92% water offer the best value for you:

1. Cucumber (96%): If you like to crunch, you're in luck. Cucumbers are the only solid food with the highest water content.

2. Iceberg Lettuce (96%) Darker greens do contain more fiber, folate, and vitamin K, but crispy iceberg is better for keeping you hydrated.

3. Celery (95%)
As well as being brimming with water, celery is an incredible wellspring of fiber. A healthy snack that also quenches thirst is made with protein-rich nut butter.

4. Radishes (95 percent) This low-calorie root vegetable is full of flavor, vitamin C, and fiber. Grate them into a summer slaw or add them to a green salad.

5. Romaine Lettuce (95 percent) This dark leafy green contains a lot of water and offers numerous nutritional advantages. Folate, vitamins C and A, and fiber are all found in abundance in romaine.

6. Tomatoes (94 percent) Despite the fact that tomatoes are the fruit with the highest water content, many people mistake them for vegetables. They also have lycopene, which protects cells from damage.

7. Zucchini and summer squash (94 percent) Summer squash contains the same amount of water whether it is cooked or raw. So make it a point to toss a few zucchini on the barbecue close to your turkey burger.

8. Asparagus (92 percent) Most people prefer to eat cooked asparagus because of its rough texture. However, since its water content remains the same whether it is cooked or eaten raw, you can grill some spears.

9. Bell peppers (92 percent) All colors of bell peppers can quench your thirst, but the ones that are green contain the most water. Bell peppers contain a lot of antioxidants, which is a bonus.

10. Cabbage (92 percent) All common varieties of cabbage contain a significant amount of water when cooked and raw. A few Chinese cabbages, for example, bok choy, are 96% water and taste incredible prepared into a plate of mixed greens.

11. Cauliflower (92 percent) You're in luck if you like riced cauliflower but don't like it raw. Like cabbage, cooked cauliflower contains 93% more water than raw cauliflower.

12. Mushrooms (92%) Mushrooms have impressive health benefits. However, consume your mushrooms raw to get the most water out of them.

13. Spinach (92 percent) Spinach is an excellent summertime addition to smoothies and salads. It is packed with nutrition, including calcium, magnesium, iron, and potassium, in addition to its high water content.

14. Strawberries (92 percent) These sour berries are a great option when you're hot and sweating a lot. They are low in calories but high in vitamin C, water, and fiber. Watermelon (92%) It goes without saying that watermelon will keep you hydrated. However, like tomatoes and other red vegetables and fruits, it also contains a lot of lycopene.

Hydration Helpers

You'll be well on your way to happy hydration if you use these seven methods!

1. Oatmeal makes a great breakfast. The classic is this one. Oatmeal is not only filling and hearty, but it also helps you stay hydrated. At the point when oats are cooking, they grow and assimilate the water or milk they're being matched with. Not into warm morning meals when it's blistering out? Attempt for the time being oats. Overnight oats have all the benefits of hot oatmeal without the heat when served cold. When making your overnight oats, sprinkle chia seeds on top.

These seeds absorb ten times their weight in extra liquid and keep you full all morning.

2. Add additional moo. Due to its source of protein, carbohydrates, calcium, and electrolytes, milk is more hydrating than water or sports drinks, according to a McMaster University study3.

3. Attempt carb options. When planning meals, avoid dry, high-carb staples like pasta. Choose zucchini noodles, also known as zoodles, which can contain approximately 95% water. This dish has the potential to deliver a hydrating and healthy punch when served with tomato sauce, which typically contains approximately 90% water.

4. Have a smoothie. Smoothies are a great and tasty way to stay hydrated thanks to the yogurt and all the fresh fruit. Not certain what products of the soil to pick? Peaches, spinach, blueberries, strawberries, and cucumbers are all excellent choices.

5. Load your plate with vegetables. Salads, like smoothies, are a great way to hydrate yourself. Even

before adding other vegetables, the majority of lettuce greens contain at least 94% water. Include carrots, bell peppers, celery, and tomatoes in your next salad.

6. Suck on soup. Gazpacho or soups made with broth are great options for satisfying and hydrating meals when you're in the mood for one. Gazpacho doesn't make you sweat in the summer when it's served cold. This filling soup is made by combining cucumbers, bell peppers, tomatoes, onions, and garlic cloves.

7. Fruit can be frozen. Are you thinking back to the popsicles you used to like as a kid? Reintroduce this timeless dessert as a delectable means of rehydrating. Fill Popsicle molds with a hydrating ingredient like watermelon, blend, and freeze for one hour.

Chapter 2
Follow a balanced Diet

We sometimes eat for the pleasure of trying new foods and enjoying their flavors. Sharing food and feasts are significant get-togethers.

However, other than for pleasure, we require food for energy, vitamins, and nutrients.

Not many food sources are either completely fine or all awful. It should be easier to eat well and enjoy food if you know how to balance your diet.

A healthy diet requires seven essential components: water, vitamins, minerals, carbs, protein, fat, fiber, and fat.

According to Maruschak, a kidney-friendly diet should focus on fruits, vegetables, whole grains, low-fat dairy, and lean meats like seafood, poultry, eggs, legumes, nuts, seeds, and soy products instead of sodium, cholesterol, and fat. She adds that individuals who have already been diagnosed with CKD might also need to restrict certain other nutrients.

For kidney health, eating a well-balanced diet is essential. Here are some suggestions to get you started:

Restrict sodium: A high sodium intake can harm your kidneys by causing fluid retention and raising blood pressure. Fresh, unprocessed foods should be preferred over processed ones as much as possible.

Boost potassium: Potassium can help lower blood pressure by counteracting the negative effects of sodium. A few decent wellsprings of potassium incorporate bananas, oranges, spinach, yams, and avocados.

Monitor Protein Consumption: While protein is significant for keeping up with bulk, consuming an excess of protein can overburden the kidneys. Choose high-quality protein sources like lean meats, fish, eggs, and plant-based sources like legumes and nuts for a moderate protein intake.

Keep hydrated: Kidney health depends on drinking enough water. Unless otherwise directed by your healthcare provider, aim for eight cups of water per day.

Contain Phosphorus: Kidney damage can result from too much phosphorus. Reduce your intake of phosphorus-rich foods like cheese, processed meats, and carbonated beverages.

Select wholesome fats: Avoid saturated and trans fats, which can make you more likely to get heart disease and damage to your kidneys. Instead, opt for fats that are good for you, like olive oil, nuts, seeds, and fatty fish.

Control Glucose: Preventing kidney damage requires controlling your blood sugar levels if you have diabetes. For diabetes management, adhere to the recommendations of your healthcare provider.

Remember that you should always talk to a doctor, especially a registered dietitian, before making major changes to your diet.

 Maintaining good kidney health requires eating a balanced diet. The kidneys are liable for sifting byproducts and overabundance liquids from the blood, so supporting their capability with a sound diet is fundamental. For kidney health, a variety of nutrient-dense foods in appropriate portions are part of a balanced diet.

Limiting sodium intake is one of the primary guidelines for a healthy diet for the kidneys. Too much sodium can cause fluid retention and kidney damage, both of which can raise blood pressure. Consuming fresh, unprocessed foods as much as possible and limiting or avoiding processed foods is the best way to reduce sodium intake.

Increasing potassium intake is another important aspect of a healthy diet for the kidneys. Potassium can assist with checking the adverse consequences of sodium on pulse. Avocados, bananas, spinach, sweet potatoes, and other fruits and vegetables are all excellent sources of potassium.

Additionally, consuming protein in moderation is essential for kidney health. It is best to aim for a moderate intake of high-quality protein sources like lean meats, fish, eggs, and plant-based sources like legumes and nuts because too much protein can strain the kidneys.

Another essential component of a kidney-healthy diet is keeping hydrated. Individuals should aim for at least eight cups of water per day, unless their healthcare provider recommends otherwise, as drinking enough water is essential for kidney function.

Additionally, limiting phosphorus intake is essential for kidney health. It is best to avoid foods high in phosphorus, such as processed meats, cheese, and carbonated beverages, as this can damage the kidneys. Choosing healthy fats is essential for kidney health. Healthy fats like olive oil, nuts, seeds, and fatty fish are best because saturated and trans fats can increase the risk of heart disease and kidney damage.
Last but not least, controlling blood sugar is essential for avoiding kidney damage, particularly in diabetics. Following medical care supplier proposals for overseeing diabetes is basic for keeping up with kidney wellbeing.

Generally, a reasonable eating routine that remembers various supplement rich food varieties for proper segments is fundamental for keeping up with great kidney wellbeing. It is in every case best to talk with a medical services proficient, especially an enrolled dietitian, prior to rolling out huge improvements to your eating regimen.

Eating well is good for your mental and physical health.

Obesity, heart disease, diabetes, hypertension, depression, and cancer risk and severity can all be reduced by it.

Eight new ways to improve your diet to keep your kidneys healthy are listed below.

1. Portion Your Plate Maruschak recommends following the MyPlate method at every meal as a general rule: Vegetables and fruits should make up about half of your plate, lean protein should make up about 25%, and whole grains should make up the remaining 25%.

2. Limit Your Salt Admission
Sodium slips its direction into a wide range of spots you wouldn't envision, particularly bundled food varieties like soups and breads. Keeping your blood pressure under control is made easier by limiting your sodium intake. According to the Dietary Guidelines for

Americans, 2020–2025, which were released by the United States Department of Agriculture (USDA), aim for 2,300 milligrams per day, which is equivalent to approximately one teaspoon of table salt.

Maruschak recommends following a low-sodium diet, specifically the Dietary Approaches to Stop Hypertension (DASH) eating plan, if you are at risk for high blood pressure or already have it. Additionally attempt these tips to hold your sodium under tight restraints:

3.Avoid eating at restaurants and ordering takeout. According to Maruschak, items used in restaurant kitchens may contain added sodium, and salt is frequently added to food. Do your homework before you eat out. She adds that the sodium content of dishes can sometimes be found on the restaurant's website.
Cook at home with entire, natural food varieties. You have complete control over how much sodium (and fat) is in each bite when you make meals at home with fresh ingredients.
Play around with seasonings. Maruschak proposes staying away from salt while cooking or at the table. Use

herbs, spices, lemon, and other salt-free seasonings instead.

Really take a look at the bundle. High-sodium food is anything prepared with more than 20% of your recommended daily sodium intake. When you can, choose soups, frozen meals, and other packaged foods with the label "reduced," "low-sodium," or "salt-free." Before consuming, rinse cans. This helps get rid of too much sodium.

4. Keep in mind that when you eat protein, your body makes waste that your kidneys filter through. Although protein is an essential component of a healthy diet, overindulging in it may force your kidneys to work harder. As noted in a 2020 study, research on the effects of a high-protein diet on kidney health is still evolving. However, if you already have CKD, your doctor will probably recommend a lower-protein diet. According to Maruschak, excessive protein intake can result in waste accumulation in the blood, which your kidneys may not be able to eliminate.

To slow the progression of kidney disease, Maruschak recommends limiting protein intake to 0.6 to 0.8 grams per kilogram of body weight for people with any stage of CKD who are not on dialysis. According to the National Kidney Foundation of Hawaii, for instance, a person weighing 150 pounds (68 kilograms) would require 40 to 54 grams of protein per day, or 4 to 6 ounces of protein from animal or plant sources. If you want to know how much protein is right for you, talk to a registered dietitian.

Even if you haven't been told you have CKD, choosing protein from healthier sources and watching how much you eat can help. Protein-rich foods include:

Eggs Dairy (one portion of yogurt and milk is 12 cups, while one portion of cheese is 1 ounce roughly the size of your two thumbs together) Beans, chickpeas, lentils, and peas (one portion is 12 cups) Nuts (one portion is 14 cups)

 5. Lean meat, fish, or skinless poultry (one portion size is 2 to 3 ounces, or about the size of a deck of cards) Choose complex carbohydrates over simple carbohydrates Carbohydrates are your body's primary source of energy, and those that are found naturally in

fresh foods are high in fiber, which helps to maintain stable blood sugar levels and support gut and heart health. However, simple carbs, like added sugars in desserts, sweetened beverages, and many packaged foods, can raise blood sugar and increase the risk of obesity, type 2 diabetes, and cardiovascular disease.

6. Diets that are high in saturated and trans fats raise the risk of heart disease, and what's bad for your heart is also bad for your kidneys. According to Maruschak, the health of the heart and kidneys are intertwined because the heart continuously pumps blood throughout the body and the kidneys continuously filter the blood to remove waste products and excess fluid from the body.

Saturated fats should make up no more than 10% of your daily calories, according to the USDA's dietary guidelines. Principal sources incorporate meats, full-fat dairy items, spread, grease, coconut oil, and palm oil, says Maruschak. Also, try to stay away from trans fats, which are found in fried and baked goods. Instead, eat a lot of unsaturated fats, which are good for your heart and can be found in fatty fish, olives, walnuts, avocados, and other vegetable oils.

7. Maruschak explains that drinking alcohol can harm your kidneys in a number of ways. It is a waste product that your kidneys must remove from your blood and reduce their effectiveness. It dehydrates you, which can make it harder for your kidneys to keep your body's water levels in check. It may have an effect on how well your liver works, which can affect how much blood flows to the kidneys and eventually cause CKD. Additionally, drinking a lot of alcohol has been linked to an increased risk of kidney disease-causing high blood pressure.

8. Talk to your doctor about whether you should cut back on phosphorus and potassium. Your body needs phosphorus and potassium for certain processes. Potassium helps regulate your heartbeat and keeps your muscles working properly, while phosphorus helps build strong bones.

However, if you have chronic kidney disease (CKD), these minerals may accumulate in your blood and cause issues throughout your body. Phosphorus can pull calcium from your bones, making them weaker and more likely to break. It can also make your skin itch and cause pain in your bones and joints. Phosphorus-rich foods like dairy, animal protein, and dark sodas may need to be limited. Heart problems can result from high potassium levels, which are found in dairy products and some fruits and vegetables. Your potassium and phosphorus levels will be measured by your doctor through blood tests. If you are unsure whether you need to monitor your intake of these minerals, be sure to ask.

Tips to Help Prevent or Manage Chronic Kidney Disease

A solid eating regimen can assist with keeping your kidneys working appropriately.
iStock (2) The Centers for Disease Control and Prevention (CDC) estimates that more than one in seven adult Americans suffer from chronic kidney disease (CKD), but the majority of people don't realize they have the condition until it has progressed significantly.
Since late-stage kidney sickness can cause a development of waste in your body and lead to various other medical issues including gout, bone illness, and coronary illness it's smart to safeguard your kidney well

being regardless of whether you haven't been determined to have CKD.

One of the most important things you can do to prevent or treat CKD is to improve your diet. What you need to know about eating to help your kidneys is in the following.

How a person's diet can affect their kidney health The kidneys are filled with tiny blood vessels that help remove waste and extra water from the body. In the event that you have CKD, your kidneys can't channel blood along with they ought to, making overabundance squander develop in your body.

Kidney disease is primarily brought on by diabetes and hypertension, also known as high blood pressure. According to Krista Maruschak, RD, a registered dietitian at the Cleveland Clinic, high blood sugar levels and high blood pressure can damage the blood vessels of the kidneys, making it impossible for them to perform their functions properly.

According to Maruschak, untreated or uncontrolled diabetes and high blood pressure can significantly influence the progression of CKD over time.

As indicated by the CDC, 11.3 percent of the U.S. populace has diabetes and 38 percent of grown-ups have prediabetes, while about a portion of American grown-ups have hypertension. Additionally, these people are more likely to develop CKD.

According to Maruschak, a healthy diet can help you keep a healthy weight and prevent or manage conditions like diabetes and high blood pressure. Thus, this supports your kidney wellbeing.

The 20 best food for people with kidney Disease

- Cauliflower
- Red bell peppers
- Cabbage
- Onions
- Garlic
- Apples
- Cranberries
- Blueberries
- Cherries

•Red grapes
•Egg whites
•Fish
•Lean meats (chicken, turkey)
•Low-sodium canned vegetables
•Low-sodium canned soups
•Low-sodium broths
•Rice
•Pasta
•Bread
•Low-fat milk

1.Cauliflower: is a cruciferous vegetable that is wealthy in supplements and low in calories, making it an extraordinary expansion to a sound eating regimen, particularly for individuals with kidney sickness. It is a great source of vitamin C, vitamin K, folate, and fiber, all of which are important for maintaining overall health and well-being.

Cauliflower's low levels of potassium and phosphorus, two minerals that can be difficult to remove from the blood when the kidneys are not working properly, make it beneficial for people with kidney disease. The presence of high blood levels of potassium and phosphorus can result in complications like heart disease and bone disease.

Cauliflower can be delighted in various ways, including crude or cooked. It can be substituted for rice or potatoes in recipes by being roasted, steamed, or mashed. It can also be blended into smoothies or soups for flavor and nutrients.

Despite the fact that cauliflower is a nutritious food option, it should not be used as a sole treatment for kidney disease and should not be used as such. Working with a doctor or registered dietitian to create a customized meal plan that meets each person's dietary requirements and preferences is highly recommended.

2. Red bell peppers :The bright red color and sweet flavor of red bell peppers, a type of sweet pepper, make them popular in the kitchen. They are a great option for people with kidney disease because they not only add flavor to meals but also offer a variety of health benefits.

One of the vital advantages of red ringer peppers is their high content of L-ascorbic acid. Truth be told, one medium-sized red ringer pepper contains around 150% of the suggested everyday admission of L-ascorbic acid. L-ascorbic acid is a cancer prevention agent that can assist with safeguarding cells from harm brought about by destructive free extremists. This is particularly significant for individuals with kidney illness, as they are at an expanded gamble of oxidative pressure, which can harm kidney cells.

Red chime peppers are likewise a decent wellspring of vitamin A, which is significant for keeping up with sound vision and skin. Furthermore, they contain vitamin B6, which assumes a part in resistant framework capability, and potassium, which can assist with directing pulse and forestall liquid maintenance.

Red bell peppers' low potassium and phosphorus content is another important benefit for people with kidney disease. Because the kidneys may not be able to remove these minerals effectively, high blood levels of these minerals can be harmful to people with kidney disease. Red bell peppers, on the other hand, are a good option for people with kidney disease because they are low in both of these minerals.

Red bell peppers can be used in a variety of dishes, including salads, stir-fries, and roasted vegetables, and they can be eaten raw or cooked. They can also be stuffed with a variety of fillings to make a meal that tastes good and is good for you. In general, red bell peppers are a delicious and nutritious addition to a well-balanced diet, and this is especially true for people who suffer from kidney disease.

3.Cabbage: Cabbage is a leafy green vegetable in the cruciferous family, along with Brussels sprouts, broccoli, and cauliflower. It is a versatile, nutritious vegetable that can be eaten raw or cooked and has numerous health benefits, especially for kidney disease patients.

The low potassium content of cabbage is one of its main advantages for people with kidney disease. The regulation of blood pressure and the proper functioning of nerves and muscles are both aided by potassium, an essential mineral. However, potassium levels can become dangerously high when the kidneys are not working properly. Cabbage is a low-potassium vegetable that can be included in a diet that is good for the kidneys to help keep potassium levels in check.

Additionally, cabbage contains a lot of fiber, which can aid in digestion and prevent constipation. It also has vitamin C, vitamin K, and vitamin B6, as well as a small amount of calcium, magnesium, and iron, which are all important nutrients.

The potential anti-inflammatory properties of cabbage are an additional significant advantage. According to some studies, the compounds in cabbage may reduce body inflammation, which could be beneficial for people with kidney disease who are more likely to suffer from chronic inflammation.

Cabbage can be used in a variety of dishes, including salads, slaws, soups, and stews, and it can be eaten raw or cooked. It can also be fermented to make foods like sauerkraut, which can help improve your health by helping your gut bacteria grow and thrive.

In general, cabbage is a healthy vegetable that is good for the kidneys. It can be included in a well-balanced diet to help control potassium levels, improve digestive health, and supply essential vitamins and minerals.

4.Onion: In many cuisines around the world, onions are a common ingredient. They are also widely used for their medicinal properties. They belong to the Allium family, which also includes shallots, garlic, and leeks. Because of their abundance of nutrients and compounds, onions are an excellent addition to any diet, but they are especially beneficial to people with kidney disease.

Onions' high antioxidant content is one of their primary advantages. Cells are shielded from damage by harmful free radicals, which can contribute to chronic conditions like kidney disease, by antioxidants. A compound known as quercetin, which has been demonstrated to possess potent antioxidant properties, is particularly abundant in onions.

Kaempferol, a type of flavonoid found in onions, has been shown to have antimicrobial and anti-inflammatory properties. Because kidney disease frequently causes inflammation and infections, these properties may be especially beneficial to sufferers.

Additionally, onions lack the minerals potassium and phosphorus, which are essential nutrients for people with kidney disease. As a result, onions can be included in a well-balanced diet as a kidney-friendly vegetable.

Onions are a versatile ingredient that can be used in a variety of dishes, including salads, stir-fries, soups, stews, and raw food. They can also be added to pizza, burgers, and sandwiches after being caramelized to bring out their natural sweetness.

It is essential to keep in mind that onions may interact with certain medications and cause gas and bloating in some individuals. As a result, it is essential to consult a physician before significantly increasing onion consumption or taking onion supplements.

In general, onions are a flavorful and nutritious food that can help people with kidney disease by protecting them from free radicals, reducing inflammation, and having low levels of potassium and phosphorus.

5.Garlic: The herb garlic has been used for centuries as
a culinary and medicinal ingredient. It belongs to the
family of Allium, which also includes shallots, leeks,
and onions. Garlic contains a compound called allicin,
which is liable for its particular smell and large numbers
of its medical advantages.

Garlic's potential to lower blood pressure is one of its
primary advantages. A common complication of kidney
disease is high blood pressure, which can be reduced to
slow the disease's progression. Although more research
is needed to confirm this, some studies suggest that
garlic supplements may help lower blood pressure.

Additionally, garlic may have anti-inflammatory
properties, which may be beneficial to kidney disease
patients. Ongoing irritation is a typical difficulty of
kidney infection and can add to the movement of the
sickness. Garlic has compounds in it that may help the
body fight oxidative stress and reduce inflammation.

Additionally, it has been demonstrated that garlic
possesses antimicrobial properties, which can aid in the

prevention of infections. This is important for people who have kidney disease because they have a weaker immune system and are more likely to get sick.

It is essential to keep in mind that garlic may interact with some medications, including warfarin and other blood thinners. As a result, before taking garlic supplements or significantly increasing your garlic intake, it's important to talk to a doctor.

Soups, stews, sauces, and marinades are just some of the many ways that garlic can be used in cooking. It can likewise be eaten crude, in spite of the fact that it tends to be areas of strength for very flavor when eaten along these lines. Generally, garlic is a tasty and sound fixing that can be remembered for a reasonable eating routine to assist with overseeing circulatory strain, diminish irritation, and give significant antimicrobial advantages.

6. Apple: Apples are a widely consumed fruit because of their crisp texture and sweet flavor. Additionally, they are a nutritious food option with numerous health benefits, including those for kidney disease.

Apples are a good source of antioxidants, which can help reduce inflammation and prevent cell damage in the body. Additionally, apples are low in sodium and fat, and they contain approximately 95 calories, 4 grams of fiber, and 14% of the daily recommended intake of vitamin C.

For individuals with kidney sickness, apples are an extraordinary food decision since they are low in potassium, which is a significant mineral that should be painstakingly observed in the eating routine of individuals with kidney illness. A variety of symptoms, including muscle weakness, fatigue, and an irregular heartbeat, can result from high potassium levels. Thus, individuals with kidney sickness genuinely should keep away from high-potassium food varieties like bananas, oranges, and potatoes, and on second thought pick low-potassium choices like apples.

Apples are also a good source of fiber, which is good for the digestive system and can help prevent constipation, which is common in kidney disease patients. Apples also contain a lot of vitamin C, which can help strengthen the immune system and prevent infections. This is especially important for people with kidney disease, who may be more likely to get infections.

In general, apples are a nutritious and kidney-friendly food option that can be enjoyed raw, baked, or added to salads or smoothies. When selecting apples, look for fruit that is firm, unbroken, smooth, and bright in color.

7. Cranberries: Native to North America, cranberries are a type of small, tart berry. They are a common food and have been used for centuries as a medicine. Cranberries are a nutritious food that has many health benefits, especially for people with certain diseases like kidney disease.

Cranberries are an excellent source of the vitamins C and E, as well as antioxidants that aid in the body's defense against free radicals and inflammation. Flavonoids, which are substances linked to a lower risk of cardiovascular disease and some types of cancer, are also present in them.

One of the most notable medical advantages of cranberries is their capacity to assist with forestalling urinary parcel diseases (UTIs). Proanthocyanidins, which can prevent bacteria from adhering to the bladder and urinary tract walls, are the reason for this. Men's and women's risk of recurrent UTIs has been shown to be reduced by cranberries.

Because they are low in potassium, cranberries are also a good food option for people with kidney disease. Because the kidneys are unable to remove excess potassium from the body, high blood potassium levels can be harmful to people with kidney disease. People with kidney disease can help maintain safe potassium levels by choosing foods with low potassium, like cranberries.

As well as being a good food decision, cranberries are likewise flexible and can be utilized in various ways. They are frequently used in sauces, chutneys, and juices and can be eaten raw, cooked, or dried. When selecting cranberries, look for berries that are firm, brightly colored, and free of bruises or other imperfections.

8. Blueberries: Native to North America, blueberries are a type of small, dark-colored berry. They are a well-liked food that is enjoyed all over the world due to their delicious sweetness and health benefits. Blueberries are a nutritious food that has many health benefits, especially for people with certain diseases like kidney disease.

Fiber, antioxidants, and vitamins C and K are all found in abundance in blueberries. Anthocyanins, an antioxidant found in blueberries, have been shown to have anti-inflammatory properties and may aid in the prevention of diabetes, heart disease, and cancer. Additionally, the fiber in blueberries has the potential to support healthy digestion and prevent constipation, a common problem for kidney disease patients.

Blueberries' capacity to enhance cognitive function is one of their most well-known health benefits. Blueberry antioxidants have been shown in studies to improve memory and concentration, particularly in older people. Blueberries may also help lower blood pressure and make it easier for the body to use insulin. This is good news for people with kidney disease who are at risk of having diabetes and high blood pressure.

Due to their low potassium content, blueberries are also a healthy food option for people with kidney disease. Because the kidneys are unable to remove excess potassium from the body, high blood potassium levels can be harmful to people with kidney disease. People with kidney disease can help keep their potassium levels within a safe range by choosing low-potassium foods like blueberries.

As well as being a quality food decision, blueberries are likewise flexible and can be utilized in various ways. They are frequently used in smoothies, muffins, and other baked goods and can be eaten raw, cooked, or frozen. When selecting blueberries, look for berries that are firm, brightly colored, and free of bruises or other imperfections.

9.Cherries:are a type of fruit that have a flavor that is both sweet and tart. They come in sweet cherries and tart cherries, among other varieties. Cherries are a nutritious food that has many health benefits, especially for people with certain conditions like kidney disease.

Vitamin C, fiber, and antioxidants like anthocyanins, which give cherries their deep red color, can all be found in cherries. Anti-inflammatory properties of these antioxidants have been demonstrated, suggesting that they may aid in the prevention of diabetes, heart disease, and cancer. Furthermore, the fiber in cherries can assist with advancing stomach related wellbeing and forestall blockage, which is a typical issue for individuals with kidney sickness.

The ability of cherries to lessen pain and inflammation is one of their most well-known health benefits. Particularly tart cherries have been shown to help alleviate the pain and inflammation associated with gout and arthritis. This is because anthocyanins, or compounds with anti-inflammatory properties, are present.

Due to their low potassium content, cherries are also an excellent option for kidney disease patients as a food. Because the kidneys are unable to remove excess potassium from the body, high blood potassium levels can be harmful to people with kidney disease. People with kidney disease can help maintain safe potassium levels by choosing foods with low potassium levels, like cherries.

Cherries are not only a nutritious food option, but they are also adaptable and can be used in a variety of ways. They are frequently used in desserts, jams, and sauces and can be eaten raw, cooked, or dried. When selecting cherries, look for fruit that is firm, plump, and shiny on the outside. Cherry bruises and soft cherries should be avoided.

10. grapes:The flavor of red grapes, a type of fruit, is well-known all over the world for its sweetness and juicy texture. They are a quality food decision that offers a scope of medical advantages, especially for individuals with specific medical issues like kidney sickness.

Vitamins C and K, as well as antioxidants like resveratrol, quercetin, and catechins, are abundant in red grapes. These cell reinforcements have been displayed to have mitigating properties and may assist with safeguarding against infections like malignant growth, coronary illness, and diabetes. Grapes' fiber also has the potential to support healthy digestion and prevent constipation, a common problem for kidney disease patients.

Red grapes' ability to improve heart health is one of their most well-known health benefits. Red grapes' antioxidants have been shown in studies to help lower blood pressure, lower cholesterol levels, and improve circulation. People with kidney disease, who are more likely to develop cardiovascular disease, may benefit most from this.

Red grapes are likewise a decent food decision for individuals with kidney illness since they are low in potassium. Because the kidneys are unable to remove excess potassium from the body, high blood potassium levels can be harmful to people with kidney disease. By picking low-potassium food sources like red grapes, individuals with kidney sickness can assist with keeping their potassium levels inside a protected reach.

Red grapes are not only a nutritious option, but they are also adaptable and can be used in a variety of ways. They are frequently utilized in salads, smoothies, and other dishes. They can be consumed raw, cooked, or fermented into wine. When selecting red grapes, look for fruit that is firm and plump, has a deep red color, and does not have any signs of mold or spoilage.

11.whites Egg

The clear liquid portion of an egg that covers the yolk is known as the egg white. They are a quality food decision that offers a scope of medical advantages, especially for individuals with specific medical issues like kidney sickness.

High-quality protein, which is needed to build and repair muscles and other body tissues, can be found in abundance in egg whites. They are likewise low in calories and fat, pursuing them as a decent food decision for individuals who are attempting to shed pounds or deal with their cholesterol levels.

Egg whites are a good source of protein for people with kidney disease due to their low phosphorus content. Because the kidneys are unable to remove excess phosphorus from the body, people with kidney disease may be at risk from high blood phosphorus levels.

People with kidney disease can help maintain safe levels of phosphorus by choosing foods high in phosphorus, like egg whites.

Egg whites can be boiled, scrambled, or baked in a variety of ways, and they can be used in numerous recipes to add protein without adding additional calories or fat.

12.Fish: is an excellent source of protein and omega-3 fatty acids for a healthy diet. Essential for brain function, heart health, and overall well-being, omega-3 fatty acids are essential. Additionally, fish is a good source of vitamin D and mineral selenium.

Due to its low phosphorus and potassium content, fish is an excellent food choice for people with kidney disease. Because the kidneys are unable to remove excess phosphorus and potassium from the body, people with kidney disease can have dangerously high blood levels of phosphorus and potassium. People with kidney disease can assist in maintaining safe levels of phosphorus and potassium by selecting fish that contain low levels of phosphorus and potassium, such as salmon, tuna, and cod.

13.Lean meats like turkey and chicken:
Lean meats like chicken and turkey are a good source of protein and have many health benefits, especially for people with kidney disease.

High-quality protein, which is necessary for the body's development and repair of muscles and tissues, can be found in abundance in turkey and chicken. They are also low in fat, making them a good option for people trying to control their cholesterol levels or lose weight.

Because they are low in phosphorus, lean meats like chicken and turkey are a good source of protein for people with kidney disease. Because the kidneys are unable to remove excess phosphorus from the body, people with kidney disease may be at risk from high blood phosphorus levels. People with kidney disease can help maintain safe levels of phosphorus by choosing foods high in phosphorus, like lean meats.

When preparing chicken and turkey, lean cuts of meat
should be used, and salt and fat should not be added.
Barbecuing, baking, or broiling are sound cooking
strategies that can assist with keeping up with the
healthy benefit of the meat.

14.low sodium canned vegetables

Canned vegetables can be a helpful and reasonable
method for adding more foods grown from the ground to
your eating regimen. However, a lot of canned
vegetables contain a lot of sodium, which can be bad for
kidney disease patients.

Cans of vegetables with low sodium are a healthy option
that have many health benefits, especially for people
with kidney disease. They are rich in fiber, which is
essential for healthy digestion, as well as vitamins and
minerals.

Due to their low sodium content, low-sodium canned
vegetables are an excellent option for kidney disease
patients. People with kidney disease may be at risk from
high blood pressure and fluid buildup as a result of high

sodium levels in the blood. People with kidney disease can help maintain safe sodium levels by selecting low-sodium canned vegetables.

When selecting low-sodium canned vegetables, it is essential to read the nutrition label and select sodium-free products. Look for vegetables in cans that say "low sodium" or "no salt added." Additionally, before cooking, rinsing canned vegetables with water can assist in further lowering their sodium content.

15.Canned soups :a lower sodium content than regular canned soups are known as low-sodium soups. Although sodium is an essential mineral that contributes to maintaining a healthy fluid balance in the body, excessive sodium intake can be harmful to kidney disease patients.

High blood pressure, fluid buildup, and other health issues can result from high sodium levels in the blood. People with kidney disease are frequently advised to limit their sodium intake in order to avoid these issues. Low-sodium canned soups are a brilliant choice for individuals who need a fast and simple dinner without consuming a lot of sodium.

16.Low-sodium canned soups :have less sodium than regular canned soups because they are made with less or no salt added. Additionally, they are a good source of protein, fiber, vitamins, and minerals. Because they are low in calories and fat, they are a nutritious and healthy option for people who are trying to keep their cholesterol levels and weight in a healthy range.

It is essential to read the nutrition label of low-sodium canned soups before purchasing them to ensure that they are indeed low in sodium. Soups marked "low-sodium" or "no salt added" should be looked for. To stay within your daily sodium allowance, it's also a good idea to check the serving size and limit your consumption of canned soups.

Overall, low-sodium canned soups are a healthy and convenient option for kidney disease patients who want to eat a balanced diet and limit their sodium intake.

Low-sodium broths are broths in which the majority of the salt has been removed or substituted with other flavorings. As a flavor enhancer, salt is frequently added to broths, but it can be harmful to people with certain health conditions like high blood pressure or heart disease. Low-sodium broths are a great option for these people because they have the same flavor and nutrients as regular broths but don't have as much salt.

17. Rice: is a common and widely consumed staple food worldwide. It is a versatile ingredient that works well in stir-fries, salads, soups, casseroles, and other dishes. There are various sorts of rice accessible, including white, brown, dark, and wild rice. It is essential to take into consideration aspects like flavor, texture, and nutritional value when selecting rice. For example, brown rice is better for you than white rice because it is less processed and has more fiber, vitamins, and minerals in it.

18. Paster: Another staple food that is consumed frequently all over the world is pasta. It can be served with a wide variety of sauces and toppings and is

typically made from wheat flour, water, and occasionally
eggs. Pasta, like rice, can be found in a variety of forms,
including spaghetti, penne, fettuccine, and lasagna
noodles. It is essential to take into consideration aspects
like flavor, texture, and nutritional value when selecting
pasta. White pasta is not as healthy as whole wheat pasta
because it has more nutrients and fiber and is less
processed.

19. Bread : is a common staple food all over the world.
It can be baked in a variety of shapes and sizes and is
typically made from flour, water, yeast, and salt. Bread
comes in many varieties, including white bread, whole
wheat bread, sourdough bread, and rye bread, just like
pasta and rice. It is essential to take into consideration
aspects like flavor, texture, and nutritional content when
selecting bread. White bread is not as healthy as whole
wheat bread because it has more nutrients and fiber and
is less processed.

20.Low fat Milk: that has had much of its fat removed
is known as low-fat milk. Compared to whole milk,
which contains approximately 3.5% fat, it typically has a
fat content of around 1% to 2%. If you're trying to cut

back on calories or saturated fat, low-fat milk is a great option. It has fewer calories and less fat than whole milk, but it has the same amount of calcium and other nutrients. Smoothies, soups, and baked goods are just a few of the many recipes that can be made with low-fat milk.

Chapter 3
EXERCISE REGULARLY

Kidney disease is a dangerous disease that affects millions of people around the world. This can lead to many complications, including high blood pressure, anemia, and bone disease. However, one of the most effective ways to treat kidney disease and improve your performance is to exercise regularly. In this chapter, we look at the importance and types of exercise for kidney disease and how they can help prevent and treat kidney disease. Benefits of exercise for kidney disease. Regular exercise has many benefits for people with kidney disease. Here are some ways exercise can help you manage the condition:

•Lowers blood pressure: High blood pressure is a common complication of kidney disease. However, exercise can help lower blood pressure by improving blood vessel function and reducing hardening of the arteries.

•Helps control blood sugar: Diabetes is a major risk factor for kidney disease, and people with diabetes are more likely to develop kidney disease. Exercise can help control blood sugar, reduce your risk of developing diabetes, and manage existing diabetes.

•Improve heart health. Kidney disease can put a lot of strain on the heart. Exercise can improve heart health by reducing your risk of heart disease, improving circulation, and reducing your risk of heart attack and stroke.

•Reduce inflammation: Inflammation is a common symptom of kidney disease. Regular exercise can help reduce inflammation in the body, improve overall health, and reduce the risk of complications.

•Improves muscle function: People with kidney disease often experience muscle weakness and emaciation. Regular exercise improves muscle function and reduces the risk of falls and injury.

•weight control. Exercise can help people with kidney disease maintain a healthy weight, which can be important for overall health and well-being.

•Improve bone health. Exercise can help improve bone density and reduce the risk of osteoporosis, which can be problematic for people with kidney disease. Improves mental health: Exercise has been shown to improve mood, reduce stress and improve mental health, which can be important for people with kidney disease who may be depressed and worried.

•Increases energy and stamina: Regular exercise can help increase energy levels and stamina, which can be beneficial for people with kidney disease, who may feel tired and weak. Better quality of life: Regular exercise can improve overall health and well-being, leading to a better quality of life for people with kidney disease.

Types of exercises for kidney disease patients

There are different types of exercise that can be helpful for people with kidney disease. Here are some examples:

1.Aerobic exercise: This type of exercise includes activities that increase your heart rate, such as walking, jogging, cycling, or swimming. Aerobic exercise can help improve heart health and lower blood pressure. Strength training: This type of exercise involves using kettlebells or resistance bands to strengthen your muscles. Strength training can help improve muscle function and reduce the risk of falls and injury.

2.Yoga: These types of exercises focus on flexible movements, stretching, and breathing techniques. They can help improve flexibility, reduce stress, and improve overall health.

 3.Walking: This is a low-impact exercise that can be done almost anywhere. Walking can help improve heart health, lower blood pressure and improve muscle function. Note when exercising it is important to take some precautions when playing sports with kidney disease.

4.Cycling: Cycling is another low-impact exercise that can help improve cardiovascular health and strengthen leg muscles. It can also be a fun and enjoyable outdoor activity.

5.Tai Chi: Tai chi is a gentle form of exercise that focuses on slow, rhythmic movements. It can help improve balance, flexibility, and strength, and can also be helpful in reducing stress and improving mental health.

6.Strength training. Strength training, such as lifting weights or using resistance bands, can help improve muscle strength and function. It may also be helpful in maintaining bone health.

7.Stretching: Stretching is important for maintaining flexibility and preventing injury. It can also help improve circulation and reduce stress.

some tips to keep in mind:

It is important for people with kidney disease to consult a doctor before starting a new exercise program, as some exercises may need to be modified or avoided depending on the situation. specific status of each individual.

1.Talk to your doctor: It's important to talk to your doctor before starting any exercise program. They can help you determine what type of exercise is safe for you and create a workout plan that's right for your needs.

2.Start slowly: If you're new to exercise or haven't played a sport in a while, it's important to start slowly and gradually increase the intensity and duration of your workouts. Fluid retention: Kidney disease can affect your body's ability to regulate fluids. It's important to stay hydrated before, during, and after a workout to stay hydrated.

3. Listen to your body: If you experience pain, discomfort, or shortness of breath while exercising, it's important to stop and rest.

Chapter 4

Manage your Blood pressure

Blood pressure monitoring measures the amount of pressure that blood exerts on the artery walls as the heart pumps blood around the body. This is an important indicator of heart health and can help detect potential problems such as hypertension (high blood pressure), hypotension (low blood pressure), or other cardiovascular conditions.

To monitor blood pressure, a healthcare professional or patient can use a blood pressure monitor, which consists of a cuff in the arm or wrist and an electronic device that measures blood pressure. This device can be either a manual sphygmomanometer, which includes inflating with a hand pump and using a stethoscope to listen to the blood flow, or an automatic digital monitor, which automatically measures pressure and displays results read on the screen.

Blood pressure readings are usually written as two numbers: systolic (top number) and diastolic (bottom number). Systolic pressure is the force exerted by the blood on the artery walls when the heart contracts, while diastolic pressure represents the force when the heart rests between beats.

A normal blood pressure reading is usually around 120/80 mmHg. Female. (millimeters of mercury) or less. Hypertension is defined as a constant blood pressure above 130/80 mmHg, while hypotension is defined as a constant blood pressure below 90/60 mmHg. However, blood pressure readings can fluctuate throughout the day and can be influenced by factors such as stress, physical activity, and medications.

Regular blood pressure monitoring is important for people with a family history of cardiovascular risk factors such as obesity, diabetes, or high blood pressure, and for people who have been diagnosed with high blood pressure. hypertension or other cardiovascular disease. Accurate and consistent monitoring can help healthcare professionals make informed decisions about treatment options and lifestyle changes to improve heart health.

Controlling blood pressure is an important part of kidney disease treatment because high blood pressure can worsen kidney damage and increase your risk of heart disease. Here are some solutions to help control blood pressure in kidney disease:

Tips to manage blood pressure

1.Be healthy in your weight or Maintain a healthy weight:

 Being overweight or hefty can come down on your heart, prompting hypertension. Blood pressure can be reduced by losing weight through a healthy diet and regular exercise.

2.Diet: refers to the type of food and drink that a person consumes on a regular basis. A diet can be described as a set of guidelines or rules that govern what a person eats and drinks. A healthy and balanced diet is essential for good health and preventing disease. A healthy diet should include a variety of nutrient-dense foods such as fruits, vegetables, whole grains, lean proteins, and healthy fats. These foods contain essential nutrients such as vitamins, minerals, fiber, and protein that are important for maintaining optimal health. It's also important to limit your intake of processed and high-calorie foods, as they can contribute to weight gain and increase your risk of chronic disease.

There are different types of diets that people can follow depending on their health goals, cultural or religious beliefs, personal preferences, or health conditions. Some examples of popular diets include the Mediterranean diet, vegetarian or vegan diets, low-carb diets, and intermittent fasting.

It's important to remember that a healthy diet isn't just about what you eat, but how much you eat and how you prepare it. Portion control and cooking methods can greatly affect the nutritional value of a meal. Also, staying hydrated by drinking enough water is important for maintaining a healthy diet and overall health. Therefore, a healthy diet is an important component of overall health and well-being. It involves eating a variety of nutrient-dense foods in appropriate portions while limiting processed and high-calorie foods.

3.Reducing Stress : this can be defined as the body's physiological and psychological response to demands and challenges. It is the body's natural response to prepare us to face a threat or danger. However, when stress becomes chronic or excessive, it can take a toll on our physical and mental health. Stress reduction involves taking steps to manage and minimize the factors that contribute to stress. Here are some ways to reduce stress:

4. Practice relaxation techniques. There are many different relaxation techniques that can help relieve stress, such as deep breathing, meditation, gradual muscle relaxation, and visualization. Exercise regularly: Exercise can help reduce stress by releasing endorphins, which are natural mood-enhancing chemicals. It also helps to improve overall health and reduce the risk of developing chronic diseases. Get enough sleep: Getting enough sleep is essential to managing stress. Lack of sleep can lead to increased levels of the stress hormone cortisol and can also contribute to anxiety and depression. Eat a healthy diet: A healthy and balanced diet can help reduce stress by providing your body with

essential nutrients that support your immune system and strengthen your immune system. overall health.
Do what you like. Activities you enjoy can help reduce stress by creating a feeling of well-being and relaxation. Connect with others: Social support can help reduce stress by providing a sense of belonging and emotional support.

5. Effective Time Management: Poor time management can increase stress levels. Effective time management involves prioritizing tasks and allocating time properly.
Seek professional help: If your stress becomes unbearable or interferes with your daily activities, you may need professional help from a therapist or counselor. By taking these steps to reduce stress, you can improve your overall health and lead a more fulfilling life.

chapter 5

Quit smoking

In both developed and developing nations, smoking is the most significant and preventable cause of morbidity and premature death. Over the course of the past four decades, the overall smoking rate in the United States has steadily decreased, transforming the habit from a cultural icon to a target of social exclusion. A few states have made a strong move to safeguard inhabitants from the notable and widely reported unfavorable impacts of utilizing tobacco items. Smoking prevalence rates range from a high of nearly 30% in Kentucky and West Virginia to a low of less than 13% in California and 10% in Utah [1]. Since smoking regulations are a local matter, there is a lot of variation between states. In spite of these achievements in public health, smoking rates have plateaued over the past five years. As a matter of fact, as per the Communities for Infectious prevention and Counteraction (CDC), one out of five Americans actually illuminates consistently. 5 million fewer people would smoke if all states had programs like those in California and Utah.

However, the cigarette industry continues to thrive in other parts of the world despite extensive efforts to reduce smoking in the United States and parts of the European Union. Every day, between 80,000 and 100,000 children start smoking around the world. Smoking will result in the deaths of approximately 25% of children in the Asia-Pacific Region [3]. These alarming figures don't just affect our international neighbors; rather, because of the rising number of immigrants arriving in the United States each year, they have a direct impact on the health care system there. The patterns in mortality for the six driving reasons for death in the US have been steady or diminishing, save one: COPD, or chronic obstructive pulmonary disease

The percentages of deaths from heart disease, stroke, and accidents decreased the most between 1970 and 2002, ranging from 40 to 60 percent. COPD death rates, on the other hand, doubled during those years [4]. Smokers and ex-smokers are catching up to the legacy of our romanticization of cigarettes throughout the majority of the 20th century as they age and develop more health issues. Those who started smoking cigarettes decades ago, when smoking was less regulated, are represented by the skyrocketing COPD rates we see today. Recent victories in anti smoking legislation are not expected to have an effect on the rate of COPD for some time.

The World Health Organization says that smokers are more likely to get:

Cellular breakdown in the lungs
Bladder malignant growth
Lung illness
Mouth malignant growth
Coronary illness
Pancreas malignant growth
Hypertension
Cervical malignant growth
Stroke
Pregnancy difficulties
Kidney malignant growth
Early menopause

Cellular breakdown in the lungs outline

Cellular breakdown in the lungs is a threatening growth that creates in the cells of the lungs. It is one of the most widely recognized sorts of disease overall and is liable for countless malignant growth related passes. Lung cancer can be divided into two categories: Lung cancer with small cells and non-small cells. The most prevalent type is non-small cell lung cancer, which accounts for approximately 85% of all cases. Lung cancer with small cells is less common than non-small cell lung cancer, but it tends to grow and spread more quickly.

Because tobacco smoke contains numerous chemicals that can harm lung cells and raise the risk of developing cancer, lung cancer is frequently linked to smoking. However, other factors, such as exposure to secondhand smoke, air pollution, and genetics, can also cause nonsmokers to develop lung cancer.

A persistent cough, chest pain, shortness of breath, wheezing, bloody coughing, fatigue, unexplained weight loss, and loss of appetite are all signs of lung cancer. However, lung cancer may not manifest any symptoms until it has progressed to a later stage in some instances.

Lung cancer treatment is determined by the patient's overall health as well as the type and stage of the disease. Therapy choices might incorporate a medical procedure, radiation treatment, chemotherapy, designated treatment, and immunotherapy. A combination of these treatments may be utilized in some instances.

Lung cancer is unfortunately difficult to treat, especially if it has spread to other parts of the body. The patient's age, overall health, and the extent to which the cancer responds to treatment all play a role in determining the patient's lung cancer prognosis. Early identification and treatment can work on the possibilities of effective treatment and long haul endurance.

An Overview of Bladder Cancer.

The cells of the bladder, a hollow organ in the lower abdomen that stores urine, are where bladder cancer begins. It occurs when bladder cells begin to grow out of control and form a tumor. There are several distinct types of bladder cancer, including urothelial carcinoma, squamous cell carcinoma, and adenocarcinoma.

Urothelial carcinoma, which begins in the cells that line the inside of the bladder, is the most common type of bladder cancer. Adenocarcinoma and squamous cell carcinoma are less common types that originate in the cells of the bladder that produce mucus or those cells that develop in response to chronic irritation and inflammation.

Because it can cause visible symptoms like blood in the urine, pain when urinating, or frequent urination, bladder cancer is often detected in its early stages. However, in some cases of bladder cancer, the disease may not manifest itself until it has advanced to a more advanced stage.

A family history of bladder cancer, exposure to certain chemicals like those found in the workplace, smoking, and a history of bladder infections are all risk factors for bladder cancer. Additionally, men are more likely than women to develop bladder cancer.

Surgery, chemotherapy, and radiation therapy—or a combination of these treatments—may be used to treat bladder cancer. The stage and severity of the cancer, the patient's overall health, and other individual factors all influence the choice of treatment.

After treatment, bladder cancer may recur in some cases; consequently, regular monitoring and follow-up care are essential. Imaging tests, other diagnostic tests, and routine cystoscopies (a procedure that allows doctors to look inside the bladder) are all examples of this.

The stage and grade of the cancer at the time of diagnosis, as well as the patient's overall health and response to treatment, influence the overall prognosis for bladder cancer. Treatment and early detection can increase the likelihood of a successful outcome.

Overview of Lung Disease.

The term "lung disease" encompasses a wide range of conditions that affect the lungs, including infections, inflammation, and tissue damage. Coughing, wheezing, shortness of breath, chest pain, and fatigue are just a few of the many symptoms that can be brought on by these diseases. The following are some of the most prevalent forms of lung disease:

Asthma: A constant condition wherein the aviation routes become kindled and restricted, making it challenging to relax. Allergens, exercise, cold air, stress, and other factors can all contribute to the onset of asthma symptoms, which can be mild to severe.

pulmonary obstructive disease (COPD): a group of lung conditions that progress over time, including emphysema and chronic bronchitis. Long-term exposure to cigarette smoke, air pollution, or other irritants is typically the cause of COPD, which can manifest as shortness of breath, coughing, and wheezing.

Pneumonia: a bacterial, viral, or fungal infection of the lungs. Fever, coughing, pain in the chest, and difficulty breathing are all symptoms of pneumonia.

Fibrosis of the lungs: A condition wherein the lung tissue becomes scarred and thickened, making it hard for the lungs to appropriately work. A number of things can lead to pulmonary fibrosis, such as being exposed to toxins, taking certain medications, or having an autoimmune disorder.

Cellular breakdown in the lungs: a form of lung cancer that grows in the tissue. Coughing, chest pain, and shortness of breath are all symptoms of lung cancer, which is frequently brought on by prolonged smoking.

Hypertension in the lungs: a condition in which the blood vessels in the lungs narrow, resulting in elevated lung blood pressure. The symptoms of pulmonary hypertension include fatigue, chest pain, and fainting.

Treatment for lung illness will rely upon the particular kind of infection and the seriousness of the condition. Medication, oxygen therapy, pulmonary rehabilitation, and surgery are all options for treatment. Lung disease management can often benefit from lifestyle changes like quitting smoking, eating a healthy diet, and exercising frequently.

Overview of heart cancer

Heart cancer, also called cardiac tumors, can be primary or secondary. Secondary heart cancer is cancer that has spread to the heart from another part of the body, whereas primary heart cancer is cancer that originates in the heart itself. Compared to primary heart cancer, secondary heart cancer occurs much more frequently.

The location and size of the tumor can influence the symptoms of heart cancer. There may be no symptoms at all in some instances. However, some of the most frequent signs of heart cancer include:

The causes of heart cancer are unknown, but symptoms include chest pain, shortness of breath, fatigue, irregular heartbeat, swelling of the legs, ankles, or feet, fainting, or dizziness. Certain genetic disorders, like tuberous sclerosis, and exposure to certain chemicals, like vinyl chloride, may raise the risk of developing heart cancer.

Because the signs and symptoms of heart conditions can be the same, it can be hard to tell if you have heart cancer. Echocardiograms, electrocardiograms, computed tomography (CT) scans, and magnetic resonance imaging (MRI) scans are some of the tests that can be used to diagnose heart cancer.

The patient's overall health, as well as the size, location, and type of the tumor, will all play a role in the course of treatment for heart cancer. Heart cancer is mostly treated with surgery to remove the tumor. However, chemotherapy or radiation therapy may also be utilized in some instances. A heart transplant may be required in some instances.

It's important to remember that heart cancer is so uncommon that it can be hard to find doctors who know how to treat it. If you or someone you know has been diagnosed with heart cancer, it may be beneficial to seek treatment at a specialized medical center that specializes in the treatment of this uncommon condition.

Kidney Malignant growth Outline

Kidney malignant growth, otherwise called renal cell carcinoma, is a kind of disease that structures in the phones of the kidneys. On either side of the spine in the lower back are the kidneys, which are two organs in the shape of beans. Urine is produced by them as they remove waste and excess fluids from the blood and send it to the bladder.

When cells in the kidneys grow out of control and form a mass or tumor, this is kidney cancer. There are a few different kinds of kidney cancer, but renal cell carcinoma is the most prevalent one. Transitional cell carcinoma, Wilms tumor, and renal sarcoma are other types of kidney cancer, but they are much less common.

Smoking, obesity, high blood pressure, exposure to certain chemicals or substances, a history of kidney cancer in the family, and certain genetic conditions like von Hippel-Lindau disease or hereditary papillary renal cell carcinoma are all risk factors for kidney cancer.

Side effects of kidney disease might include blood for the pee, a bump or mass in the midsection, torment in the side or lower back, weight reduction, weariness, and fever.

Surgery to remove the affected kidney or part of it, as well as any nearby lymph nodes or other tissue that may contain cancer cells, is typically the treatment for kidney cancer. Depending on the stage and severity of the cancer, additional treatments may include targeted therapy, immunotherapy, or radiation therapy.

The prognosis for kidney cancer varies based on the stage of the disease at the time of diagnosis and other factors like age and overall health. Kidney cancer can frequently be successfully treated and has a high rate of survival if discovered early. However, the prognosis may be less favorable if the cancer has spread to other parts of the body.

People at higher risk for kidney cancer should get checked and screened on a regular basis because early detection and treatment can improve outcomes.

Kidney disease and smoking.

Smoking is a significant risk factor for a number of chronic conditions, including CKD. The kidneys are in charge of removing waste products and excess fluid from the blood. If they become damaged, they may not work as well as they should. Smoking can worsen kidney disease and cause damage to the kidneys.

For kidney disease patients, smoking can be harmful in the following ways:

Reduced Flow of Blood to the Kidneys: Smoking can diminish bloodstream to the kidneys, which can prompt diminished kidney capability. The kidneys may not be able to adequately remove waste products and excess fluid from the blood if there is insufficient blood flow to them.

Kidney disease is more likely: Several chronic diseases, including diabetes and hypertension, are known to be linked to smoking. Kidney disease can be brought on by either of these conditions. As a matter of fact, diabetes and hypertension are the two driving reasons for kidney sickness in the US.

Risk of Kidney Failure at a Higher Level: Additionally, smoking can raise the likelihood of kidney failure. When the kidneys are unable to remove waste products and excess fluid from the blood in an adequate manner, this condition is known as kidney failure. Dialysis or a kidney transplant may be required to maintain life in this situation.

Extinction of the Kidney Disease: Smoking can deteriorate existing kidney sickness. Smoking, for instance, has been linked to an increase in proteinuria—a condition in which protein is found in the urine. Proteinuria is a sign of kidney damage, and if left untreated, it can cause more kidney damage.

Impedance with Prescriptions: Smoking can disrupt prescriptions that are utilized to treat kidney infection. Smoking, for instance, can make blood pressure medications less effective, which are commonly used to treat hypertension in kidney disease patients. Controlling blood pressure may become more difficult as a result, which could cause kidney damage to worsen.

In rundown, smoking is hazardous for kidney illness patients since it can diminish bloodstream to the kidneys, increase the gamble of kidney sickness and kidney disappointment, deteriorate existing kidney infection, and impede drugs used to treat kidney illness. To protect your kidneys and improve your overall health, quitting smoking is essential if you have kidney disease.

the negative effects of smoking.

Smoking can have a number of negative effects on your health, and there are a lot of potential health issues that can arise from smoking. The most serious health consequences of smoking are as follows:

1.Lung cancer: Lung cancer is most commonly caused by smoking. As indicated by the American Malignant growth Society, around 85% of cellular breakdown in the lungs cases are brought about by smoking. Other types of cancer, including mouth, throat, esophageal, bladder, kidney, and pancreatic cancer, are also more likely to be caused by smoking.

2. Problems with the airways: Smoking can cause a scope of respiratory issues, including constant bronchitis, emphysema, and asthma. Coughing, wheezing, shortness of breath, and difficulty breathing are all symptoms of these conditions.

3. Diseases of the heart: Cardiovascular disease, including heart attack, stroke, and peripheral vascular disease, is strongly correlated with smoking. Atherosclerosis, or hardening of the arteries, is a condition that can result from smoking's damage to the blood vessels. This can expand the gamble of blood clusters, which can cause coronary failures and strokes.

4. Problems with reproduction: Smoking can result in infertility, complications during pregnancy, and premature birth. Smoking during pregnancy can make a woman more likely to have a stillbirth, SIDS, or a low birth weight baby.

5. Probleme with oral health: Tooth decay, gum disease, oral cancer, and bad breath are just a few of the oral health issues that smoking can cause.

6. Vision issues: Smoking can make cataracts and age-related macular degeneration, both of which can cause blindness, more likely to happen.

8. Skin issues: Smoking can harm the skin and increase the risk of skin cancer, wrinkles, and premature aging.

Smoking can also affect your sense of taste and smell, make it harder to exercise and do physical activities, and make you more likely to have mental health issues like depression and anxiety, in addition to the aforementioned health issues.

In general, smoking is a highly risky habit that can have significant and lasting health effects. The best thing you can do for your health is to stop smoking.

Steps of Quitting Smoking

Although quitting smoking can be difficult, the benefits to your overall health and well-being are undeniable. The following are twenty steps to help you quit smoking:

1.Set a quitting date and decide to stop smoking.

2. Tell your family, companions, and associates that you're stopping smoking.

3. Plan to avoid the things that make you smoke, like stress or social situations, in the future.

4. To assist you in quitting, think about nicotine replacement therapy, such as gum or patches.

5. Converse with your PCP about physician recommended meds that can assist with smoking discontinuance.

6. To assist you in quitting, look for a counseling program or support group.

7. Manage stress and cravings by developing healthy coping mechanisms like exercise, meditation, or hobbies.

8. Get rid of anything related to smoking from your home, car, and place of employment.

9.Avoid establishments like casinos and bars where smoking is permitted.

10. Identify and alter any smoking-related routines or practices.

11. To bolster your decision to quit smoking, use positive self-talk and affirmations.

12. Reward yourself when you reach milestones on your journey to quit smoking.

13. To assist in the elimination of toxins from your body, consume healthy foods and drink a lot of water.

14. To help manage stress and cravings, get plenty of sleep and rest.

15. Avoid caffeine and alcohol, which can make you want to smoke more.

16. You can distract yourself from cravings by doing things like reading or going for a walk.

17. For stress management, try deep breathing or other relaxation techniques.

18. To assist you in quitting smoking, think about alternative treatments like hypnotherapy or acupuncture.

19. Remind yourself of the advantages of quitting smoking to maintain your motivation and focus on achieving your objectives.

20. Don't give up if you relapse; instead, take what you learned from it and use it to keep working toward a smoke-free life.

People experience the following health benefits shortly after quitting, which can significantly improve their

quality of life and serve as reminders of the potential
health benefits of quitting:

When a person stops smoking, the benefits begin to
accumulate. Breathing becomes easier on a daily basis,
coughing and wheezing become less frequent, then
disappear, and the senses of taste and smell improve.
Clearer skin, better oral health, hormone stability, a
stronger immune system, and a lower risk of a variety of
cancers are among these benefits.

benefits of quitting smoking

1. Between 20 and 12 hours later: The blood levels of
carbon monoxide and heart rate return to normal.

2. Following 1 year: Blood pressure and the risk of a
heart attack are both significantly lower. Upper
respiratory issues and coughing begin to get better.

3. In two to five years:
The gamble of stroke drops to that of somebody who
doesn't smoke, as per the CDCTrusted Source.

4. 5 to 15 years later: The risk of bladder, mouth, esophagus, and throat cancer is cut in half.

5. In ten years: Lung and bladder cancer risk is half that of a person who smokes.

6. Following 15 years: The risk of heart disease is comparable to that of not smoking.

Chapter 6

Limit Alcohol

A family of organic compounds with one or more
hydroxyl (-OH) groups attached to a carbon atom is
referred to as alcohol, which is a broad term. Ethanol
(C2H5OH), which is found in alcoholic beverages like
beer, wine, and spirits, is the most prevalent type of
alcohol. When consumed in excess, alcohol can have a
number of negative effects on the body, including
altering mood, impairing judgment and coordination,
and potentially leading to addiction and other health
issues.

according to recent research. Beyond Dry, here are some
reasons why you might want to cut back. I'm sorry if this
makes you feel bad, but drinking a glass or two of wine
every night is not good for your health.

After decades of research that was sometimes
contradictory and confusing (a little alcohol is good, but
too much is bad for you; a few kinds of liquor are
preferable for you over others; simply joking, it's all
awful), the image is becoming more clear: Even a small
amount of alcohol can be harmful to one's health.

According to a study that came out in November, excessive alcohol consumption was the cause of approximately 140,000 deaths annually in the United States between the years 2015 and 2019. Acute causes included homicides, car crashes, and poisonings in about 40% of those deaths. However, the majority were the result of long-term conditions that alcohol was blamed for, such as heart disease, cancer, and liver disease.

People frequently assume that experts are referring to people who have an alcohol use disorder when they talk about the dire health consequences of excessive alcohol consumption. However, moderate drinking can also carry the same health risks as excessive drinking.

"Risk begins to go up well beneath levels where individuals would think, 'Gracious, that individual has a liquor issue,'" said Dr. Tim Naimi, overseer of the College of Victoria's Canadian Establishment for Substance Use Exploration. " Beginning at very low levels, alcohol is harmful to health.

Here's what you need to know about when and how alcohol affects your health if you want to know if you should cut back on your drinking.

How can I tell if I've had too much to drink?
The term "excessive alcohol use" technically refers to anything above the daily limits outlined in the United States Dietary Guidelines. Men consume more than two drinks per day, while women consume more than one.

There is likewise arising proof "that there are gambles even inside these levels, particularly for specific kinds of malignant growth and a few types of cardiovascular infection," said Marissa Esser, who drives the liquor program at the Places for Infectious prevention and Counteraction.
Additionally, the recommended daily limits should not be averaged over a week. To put it another way, if you don't drink Monday through Thursday but drink two or three drinks a night on the weekends, that counts as excessive consumption. Damage can result from both the total number of drinks consumed over time and the amount of alcohol in your system at any given time.

Researchers believe that the principal way liquor causes medical conditions is by harming DNA. Acetaldehyde, a chemical that is harmful to cells, is produced when alcohol is metabolized by the body. According to Dr. Esser's explanation, acetaldehyde "damages your DNA and prevents your body from repairing the damage." When your DNA is harmed, then, at that point, a cell can outgrow control and make a malignant growth cancer."

Liquor additionally makes oxidative pressure, one more type of DNA harm that can be especially destructive to the cells that line veins. Stiffened arteries caused by oxidative stress can increase blood pressure and increase the risk of coronary artery disease.

"It essentially influences DNA, and that is the reason it influences so many organ frameworks," Dr. Naimi said. Consumption on a regular basis "damages tissues over time" over a lifetime.

Due to the fact that some studies have asserted that moderate amounts of alcohol, particularly red wine, can be beneficial, the impact of alcohol on the heart is unclear. Previous research suggested that resveratrol, an antioxidant found in grapes and red wine, has heart-protective properties and that alcohol raises HDL, or "good" cholesterol.

In any case, said Mariann Piano, a teacher of nursing at Vanderbilt College, "There's been a great deal of late proof that has truly tested the thought of any sort of what we call a cardio-defensive or solid impact of liquor."

The fact that people who drink little alcohol tend to have other healthy habits like exercising, eating a lot of fruits and vegetables, and not smoking probably led people to believe that drinking little alcohol was good for the heart. Dr. Piano stated that observational studies may have incorrectly attributed the heart benefits of those behaviors to alcohol.

Recent studies have shown that people who drink a lot have a significantly higher risk of developing high blood pressure and heart disease than those who drink little. The good news is that people's blood pressure falls when they stop drinking or just cut back. Additionally, drinking alcohol has been linked to atrial fibrillation, an abnormal heart rhythm that can lead to stroke and blood clots.

Alcohol Abuse

Addiction to alcohol is the second most common type of
substance abuse in the United States, after smoking.
Some people are affected more severely than others.

At the point when a singular's drinking causes misery or
damage, that is called a liquor use jumble. An alcohol
use disorder affects 5% of adult women and 10% of
adult men. Their alcoholism causes health issues as well
as issues at home, at work, in school, or with the law.
Numerous of them no longer have control over their
drinking; Despite the serious negative effects on their
health and the loss of valued activities and relationships,
they are unable to stop or reduce their use.

It is unclear why some people drink and others don't, but
a person is more likely to drink if they have a family
history of alcohol addiction. The disorder is four times
more likely to occur in children of parents who struggle
with alcoholism.

The liver, stomach, heart, brain, and nervous system can all be seriously harmed by excessive drinking. It also raises the risk of mouth, throat, esophagus, and larynx (voice box) cancer. Women who consume a lot of alcohol are more likely to develop osteoporosis and breast cancer. Additionally, excessive drinkers may not consume enough food, leading to vitamin and mineral deficiencies.

Despite the fact that there are many dangers to drinking liquor, there likewise might be a few advantages of moderate drinking. For men, this means no more than two drinks per day, and for women, no more than one drink per day. 5 ounces of wine, 12 ounces of beer, or 112 ounces of distilled spirits with an 80 percent proof constitute a drink.) The risk of heart disease, stroke, and other circulatory diseases appears to be reduced by moderate drinking. There is proof that a modest quantity of liquor can help levels of high-thickness lipoprotein (HDL), the useful cholesterol in your blood, as well as decrease the development of plaque in veins.

How do you determine how much alcohol is safe if too much is bad but some is good? First, don't start if you

don't drink. Frequently, the benefits of drinking alcohol
outweigh the risks. On the off chance that you drink, do
as such with some restraint — something like one
beverage daily for ladies and something like two
beverages every day for men.

People who plan to drive or operate equipment that
requires attention or skill, women who are trying to
conceive or are pregnant, and people who take
prescription or over-the-counter medications that can
cause drowsiness should not drink.

Additionally, alcohol can alter the toxicity and efficacy
of medications. Alcohol levels in the blood or the
negative effects of alcohol on the brain are increased by
some medications.

An alcohol abuse disorder is a serious condition that gets
worse over time. But it can be treated. Learn more about
the disease and ask your doctor for help if you or
someone you care about thinks they have an alcohol
problem.

Early side effects of a liquor misuse jumble incorporate drinking more than arranged, proceeding to drink liquor notwithstanding the worries of others, and continuous endeavors to chop down or quit drinking. A tolerance to alcohol is developed as alcohol abuse progresses. He or she must consume additional alcohol to achieve the desired state of happiness or to become inebriated.

When an individual becomes dependent on alcohol and is unable to consume it, they experience withdrawal symptoms such as headache, nausea, and fatigue.

The person may lose control as alcohol abuse gets worse because they become consumed with alcohol. He or she may experience blackouts, which are episodes in which, despite being conscious at the time, a person completely forgets what happened while drunk.

At last, character changes happen. Abusing alcohol can lead to aggressive behavior and a serious decline in one's ability to function (hold a job or maintain relationships with friends and family). People who drink a lot can have seizures, tremors, panic attacks, confusion, and hallucinations.

Alcoholism is often a problem for people who drink alone, and they often say they drink to relax or sleep better. Excessive drinkers may also drive when they shouldn't or engage in risky sexual behavior. Additionally, they are more likely to become dependent on other drugs.

How alcohol abuse affects the body Drinking too much alcohol has devastating effects on the body. Impotence, permanent nerve and brain damage (numbness or tingling sensations, imbalance, inability to coordinate movements, forgetfulness, blackouts, or problems with short-term memory), inflammation of the pancreas, and inflammation of the liver are some of the health effects of excessive alcohol consumption. The risk and severity of pneumonia and tuberculosis can also be increased by long-term alcohol abuse; harm to the heart, which can lead to heart failure; and lead to liver failure, which is known as cirrhosis.

Treating Alcohol Abuse

An individual who needs assistance for liquor fixation might be the last to acknowledge the person has an issue. Family members can get help and support from an organization like Al Anon even if the addict refuses treatment.

Family members can learn how to assist the addicted person in receiving the appropriate level of support and assistance from many similar drug and alcohol rehabilitation programs that offer counseling. A significant piece of these projects is to make the consumer liable for their way of behaving, and to assist the family with preventing protecting the consumer from the results of drinking.

Helping the drinker realize that he or she has a problem and needs help is the first step in treating alcohol abuse. Treatment for alcoholics who want to stop drinking can take place in either an outpatient setting (such as regular counseling sessions) or an inpatient program at a hospital (where the treatment is much more intensive).

The majority of treatment programs require complete abstinence from alcohol and other drugs because they view alcohol dependence as a chronic, progressive disease.

Detoxification, or supervised withdrawal from alcohol, is typically the first step in inpatient treatment. Medications are typically used to lessen the harmful effects of withdrawal, such as restlessness, agitation, hallucinations, delirium, and seizures. Alcohol withdrawal can be life-threatening in its worst form.

Therapy for liquor abuse additionally addresses the clinical and mental outcomes of liquor fixation. Health care providers educate the individual and their loved ones on the nature of addiction and assist the individual in locating constructive alternatives to alcohol use. Health care professionals also help the person deal with any related issues, like depression, stress at work, drinking-related legal issues, or troubled personal relationships.

Recovery, also known as maintaining sobriety, is a long-term process that can take many forms. Fellowship groups like Alcoholics Anonymous can be extremely beneficial at times.

Counseling on a regular basis and medication therapy may also be helpful. People who want to try a drug that helps them stop drinking might want to look into Disulfiram, also known as Antabuse. If a person drinks alcohol, disulfiram makes them feel sick because it prevents the liver from breaking down alcohol.

Naltrexone (Revia, Vivitrol) is another drug that makes people less interested in drinking because it takes away the pleasant feeling that comes with it. Acamprosate, or Campral, is a third drug that helps alcoholics feel better when they don't drink.

Alcohol and Kidney Disease.

Consuming alcohol can have a significant impact on kidney health, especially in people with kidney disease already. The kidneys are essential for removing waste from the blood and maintaining a healthy fluid balance in the body. The kidneys' normal function can be disrupted by alcohol, leading to a variety of kidney issues.

Dehydration is one of the main ways that alcohol can harm the kidneys. Alcohol is a diuretic, which means that it makes more urine, which can make you dehydrated if you don't get enough of it. Drying out can decrease the bloodstream to the kidneys and hinder their capacity to accurately work. Chronic alcohol dehydration can cause kidney damage, including the formation of kidney stones, over time.

Inflammation of the kidneys is another way alcohol can affect kidney health. Acetaldehyde, a toxic byproduct of alcohol metabolism, can build up in the kidneys from excessive drinking. Acetaldehyde can irritate the kidneys and cause scar tissue to form, both of which can affect kidney function.

Consuming alcohol can also raise blood pressure, which can damage the kidneys' blood vessels and make it harder for them to work properly. Having high blood pressure can also make it more likely that you will get kidney disease or have it get worse.

Consumption of alcoholic beverages can be particularly harmful to kidney disease patients. Reduced kidney function makes it more difficult for people with kidney disease to process alcohol. Consequently, even moderate alcohol consumption can significantly raise the risk of kidney damage and kidney disease progression.

In conclusion, drinking alcohol can have a significant impact on kidney health, particularly in people who already have kidney disease. Dehydration, inflammation, and high blood pressure caused by alcohol can all harm the kidneys and make it harder for them to work properly. To protect the kidneys and prevent further damage, people with kidney disease must abstain from alcohol or limit their intake.Alcohol Abuse

Steps to Reduce Alcohol Consumption

Determine the reasons you want to reduce alcohol consumption. This could be done to save money, improve your relationships, or improve your health. Set goals that are specific and doable. For instance, assuming you right now drink 4 beverages each evening, expect to lessen that to 2 beverages each evening.

Be aware of things that make you want to drink. These could be specific individuals, places, or activities that or practicing relaxation techniques like deep breathing could be part of this.

Get rid of alcohol in your home. You'll be less likely to drink if you don't have easy access to alcohol.

Select alternatives that are not alcoholic. At the point when you're out with companions or at a get-together, request a non-cocktail rather than a heavy drinker one. When you drink, take your time. Drink water or other non-alcoholic beverages in addition to alcoholic drinks, and sip rather than swallow.

Drinking when hungry is not a good idea. The absorption of alcohol into the bloodstream can be slowed down by eating a meal prior to drinking.

Learn to say no to pressure from others. You don't have to drink just because someone else says you should. Seek the support of friends and family who agree with your decision to cut back on alcohol consumption.

If you think you need more structured support, you might want to join a support group like Alcoholics Anonymous.

Engage in stress-relieving activities like yoga, meditation, or physical activity. Finding healthy ways to cope with stress can help reduce the urge to drink because stress can be a trigger for drinking.

Establish limits for yourself. This could mean limiting the amount of time you spend with people who make you want to drink or staying out of certain social situations entirely.

To keep track of your progress, keep a journal. Keep track of when you were successful in reducing your alcohol consumption and the methods that worked for you.

If you make a mistake, don't beat yourself up. When trying to change one's behavior, relapse is common. Instead of giving up, use it as a learning opportunity and get back on track.

Avoid "triggers" that can cause excessive drinking. Avoid situations or people that you know are likely to make you want to drink if at all possible.

Make an effort to find alcohol-free alternatives. For instance, assuming that you like the flavor of brew, take a stab at drinking non-hard lager all things being equal.

Be surrounded by people who are encouraging and supportive of your efforts to cut back on alcohol consumption.

Give yourself a reward when you reach your goals. To celebrate your success, for instance, treat yourself to a spa day or a movie night with friends.

Finally, treat yourself with patience. It takes time to change one's behavior, so be kind to yourself along the way. Keep in mind that progress is progress, regardless of how small the step may be.

Chapter 7

Get enough sleep

Sleeping enough is important for maintaining good mental and physical health. Adults should get between 7 and 9 hours of sleep each night, but this can vary from person to person.

The pace of modern life sometimes leaves you with little time to stop and rest. It can make it seem impossible to get a good night's sleep on a regular basis.

However, just as diet and exercise are essential for good health, so is sleep. Sleeping well improves mood, health, and brain function.

Not getting sufficient quality rest consistently raises the gamble of numerous infections and problems. These include obesity, dementia, heart disease, and stroke.

There's something else to great rest besides only the hours spent in bed, says Dr. Marishka Brown, a rest master at NIH. " Sound rest includes three significant things," she makes sense of. " The first is how much you sleep. Another factor is the quality of your sleep—having restful, uninterrupted sleep. The final one is a regular sleeping schedule.

It may be more difficult for people who work night shifts or on irregular schedules to get enough sleep. Additionally, periods of extreme stress, such as the current pandemic, can disrupt our normal sleeping patterns. However, there are numerous ways to improve your sleep.

Rest for Fix
For what reason do we have to rest? According to Dr. Maiken Nedergaard, a sleep researcher at the University of Rochester, people frequently misunderstand sleep as merely "down time," when a tired brain gets some rest.

She states, "But that's wrong." Your brain is working while you sleep. For instance, rest readies your mind to learn, recollect, and make.

The brain has a drainage system that removes toxins while you sleep, according to Nedergaard and her colleagues.

She explains, "The brain completely changes function when we sleep." It removes waste from the body, acting almost like a kidney.

Last night, how many hours of sleep did you get? The National Sleep Foundation updated its sleep recommendations earlier this year and states that young adults (age 18 to 25) and adults (age 26 to 64) should sleep 7 to 9 hours, but not less than 6 hours, more than 10 hours, or 11 hours (for adults) or less. Adults over 65 should get 7 to 8 hours of sleep per night, with no less than 5 hours or more than 9 hours.

Getting the recommended amount of sleep can be difficult given all of the responsibilities we have as practitioners, academics, and family members. The lack of sleep is a public health issue, according to the Centers for Disease Control and Prevention earlier this year. The importance of getting enough sleep to our health has been demonstrated by numerous studies. The National Heart, Lung, and Blood Institute says that people who don't get enough sleep are more likely to have heart disease, kidney disease, high blood pressure, diabetes, stroke, and obesity.

A lack of sleep can have a number of negative effects, including fatigue, inability to concentrate, irritability, mood swings, a weakened immune system, and an increased likelihood of accidents and injuries. Obesity, diabetes, and cardiovascular disease are some of the long-term health issues that have been linked to chronic sleep deprivation.

Ten tips for Get Enough Sleep

1.Maintain a Regular Sleep Schedule:
 Consistency is the lifeblood of your body's internal clock, also known as the circadian rhythm. Your circadian rhythm can be regulated by going to bed and

getting up at the same time every day. This can help you fall asleep faster and feel more refreshed when you wake up.
Set an alarm for both your bedtime and your wake-up time if you have trouble falling asleep or staying awake at the same time each day. This will help you stay on track with your sleep schedule. It's likewise essential to adhere to your rest plan at the end of the week, as snoozing or staying awake until late can disturb your daily schedule and make it harder to nod off the next night.

Also, try to come up with a bedtime routine that you can stick to every night, like taking a warm bath, reading a book, or listening to music that calms you down. Your body may receive a signal from this routine that it is time to wind down and prepare for sleep.

2.Make a peaceful sleeping environment:
The environment in which you sleep can have a significant impact on how well you sleep. To create a peaceful sleeping environment, follow these recommendations:

Keep your room cool, preferably between 60-67°F (15-19°C), as a cooler room temperature can advance rest.
Use earplugs or a white noise machine to block out any distracting sounds to keep your bedroom quiet.
Ensure your room is dull by utilizing power outage draperies, conceals or an eye veil. This can help you nod off and stay unconscious.
Make an investment in soft pillows and bedding. Your body should be supported in a neutral and comfortable position by your mattress and pillows.
Your bedroom should be free of electronics like laptops, phones, and televisions. Blue light from these gadgets can make it harder to fall asleep because it can stop your body from making the sleep hormone melatonin. Try activating the blue light filter or night mode on your phone if you absolutely have to have it with you.
You can help your body prepare for sleep and reduce the likelihood of disturbances that can wake you up during the night by creating a sleep environment that is comfortable and relaxing.

3 Avoid nicotine and caffeine:

Nicotine and caffeine are both stimulants that can make it hard to fall asleep and stay asleep. This is the very thing you want to be familiar with these substances: Caffeine: Caffeine, which can be found in chocolate, coffee, tea, and some medications, can stay in your system for up to eight hours after consumption. Try to avoid caffeine for at least four to six hours before going to bed in order to avoid disrupting your sleep. If you find that caffeine is having an effect on your sleep, you might want to reduce the amount you drink overall.

Nicotine: Like caffeine, nicotine is a stimulant found in tobacco products and can disrupt sleep. Smokers are more likely to wake up during the night and have more trouble sleeping. Try to completely stop smoking or don't smoke before bed to avoid the stimulating effects of nicotine.

In addition to nicotine and caffeine, try to avoid alcohol, sugary foods, large meals before bedtime, and other stimulants that can disrupt sleep. If you have to snack before going to bed, choose something light and conducive to sleep, like a banana or a small bowl of whole-grain cereal with milk.

4 Avoid alcohol before going to bed:

Even though drinking alcohol may initially induce
drowsiness and help you fall asleep more quickly, it can
actually disrupt your sleep at night. This is why:
Alcohol can disrupt the natural cycle of sleep: While
liquor can cause you to feel sluggish and assist you with
nodding off quicker, it can likewise slow down the
normal rest cycle, making you awaken much of the time
during the evening and feel less refreshed in the first part
of the day.
Alcohol can make sleep apnea worse: Liquor can loosen
up the muscles in your throat, making it more probable
for you to wheeze or experience rest apnea, a condition
in which breathing stops or becomes shallow during rest.
Dehydration can result from alcohol: Alcohol is a
diuretic, which means that it can make more urine and
make people dehydrated. Dehydration can make it
difficult to fall asleep and cause discomfort during sleep.
Avoid alcohol before bedtime or limit yourself to one or
two drinks several hours before you plan to go to sleep
to ensure a good night's sleep. To support your overall
health and well-being, it is essential to seek treatment
and assistance if you struggle with alcohol dependence
or addiction.

5. Get active often:

Customary activity can assist you with nodding off quicker and appreciate further, more relaxing rest. How to do it:

Practice controls the rest wake cycle: Your internal clock can be regulated through regular exercise, allowing you to fall asleep faster and wake up feeling more rested.

Stress and anxiety can be reduced through exercise: Endorphins are released when you exercise, which can help you feel less stressed and anxious, two things that can make it hard to fall asleep and stay asleep.

Sleep quality can be improved by exercise: Studies have demonstrated the way that ordinary activity can further develop rest quality, assisting you with feeling more refreshed and alert during the day.

Try to get at least 30 minutes of moderate exercise every day of the week to reap the benefits of exercise for sleep. Notwithstanding, it's essential to keep away from vivacious activity late at night, as it can animate the body and make it harder to nod off. Attempt to complete your exercise something like 2-3 hours before sleep time to give your body time to slow down.

6 .Establish a sleeping schedule:

Your body's internal clock can be regulated by following a regular sleep schedule, making it easier to fall asleep and feel refreshed when you wake up. How to establish a regular sleep schedule is as follows:

Every day, even on weekends, you should go to bed and wake up at the same time: When it comes to sleeping, consistency is essential. Even on weekends, when it may be tempting to sleep in or stay up late, try to adhere as closely as possible to a regular sleeping schedule.

Establish a relaxing routine before bed: Having a regular bedtime routine can help your body know it's time to go to sleep. Make an effort to wind down before going to bed by engaging in calming activities like reading, taking a warm bath, practicing meditation, or doing exercises that require deep breathing.

Limit or avoid naps to 30 minutes: Taking naps can help you catch up on sleep, but they can also make it hard to fall asleep at night. If you do nap, don't nap for more than 30 minutes at a time or too close to bedtime.

Laying out a normal rest timetable might take some time and exertion, yet it can hugely affect your general rest quality and prosperity. Be patient as your body adjusts to the new routine by adhering to your sleep schedule as closely as you possibly can, even on weekends.

7.Create an environment that encourages sleep:
Relaxation and a quicker rate of sleep can be achieved
by creating a sleep-friendly environment. How to do it:
Maintain a quiet, cool, and dark bedroom: The
environment in your bedroom can have a big effect on
how well you sleep. To ensure a peaceful, cool, and
restful sleeping environment, make sure your bedroom is
quiet.
Make an investment in a soft mattress and pillows: You
can sleep better and feel more rested if you have a soft
mattress and pillows. Make an investment in high-
quality bedding that makes you feel comfortable.
Prior to bedtime, limit screen time: Melatonin, a
hormone that helps regulate sleep, can be disrupted in
your body by blue light from electronic devices. If you
absolutely must use an electronic device before bedtime,
use a blue light filter.
Give white noise a shot: White noise, such as the sound
of a fan or a white noise machine, can help block out
other sounds and make it easier to fall asleep.
You can help your body relax and fall asleep faster by
creating a comfortable sleeping environment. This can
help you sleep more soundly throughout the night. Make

sure your bedroom is set up for a good night's sleep and keep bright lights and loud noises out of your bedroom.

8.Avoid nicotine and caffeine before going to bed:
 Nicotine and caffeine both have the potential to prevent you from falling asleep and staying asleep. How to do it: Caffeine can cause insomnia: Caffeine is a stimulant that can make it hard to fall and stay asleep. Additionally, it may make you feel more awake and alert, making it more challenging to wind down before going to bed. Sleep issues can be caused by nicotine: Nicotine is a stimulant that can make it hard to fall and stay asleep. It can likewise make you awaken during the evening and feel less refreshed toward the beginning of the day.
It is best not to consume caffeine or nicotine before going to bed in order to avoid their detrimental effects on sleep. In the event that you're a weighty caffeine or nicotine client, attempt to step by step scale back your admission over the long run to diminish the effect on your rest. All things considered, pick decaffeinated drinks or natural teas at night, and try not to smoke or utilize nicotine items before sleep time.

9. Limit liquor utilization:

Alcohol can make you feel sleepy and help you fall asleep faster, but it can also make it hard to get a good night's sleep. This is how it's done:

Sleep cycles are disrupted by alcohol: While liquor might assist you with nodding off quicker, it can likewise disturb your rest cycle, making you awaken all the more as often as possible during the evening.

Alcohol can make it hard to fall asleep: The crucial phase of the sleep cycle known as deep sleep aids in the body's repair and restoration. However, alcohol can disrupt this stage of sleep, causing you to wake up feeling less rested.

Snoring and sleep apnea can be brought on by alcohol: Alcohol can relax the muscles in your throat, making you more likely to snore and have sleep apnea, two conditions that can make it harder to sleep.

It is best to limit your alcohol intake and avoid drinking close to bedtime in order to reduce the impact of alcohol on your sleep. Try to stop drinking at least a few hours before going to bed and limit your consumption to no more than one or two drinks per day. If you have trouble sleeping after drinking, you might want to cut back or stop drinking altogether.

10. Get active on a regular basis:
You may be able to fall asleep more quickly and have better sleep if you exercise regularly. How to do it: Exercise helps you relax: Exercise can help you relax and get rid of stress and anxiety, both of which can make it hard to fall asleep.

The sleep-wake cycle is regulated by exercise: Your body's natural sleep-wake cycle can be regulated with exercise, making it easier to fall asleep and feel rested when you wake up.

Exercise can further develop rest quality: Exercise has been shown to increase the amount of time spent in deep sleep and improve the quality of sleep.

To receive the rewards of activity on rest, expect to get somewhere around 30 minutes of moderate-power practice most days of the week. However, exercising too close to bedtime can have the opposite effect and make it harder to fall asleep, so it's important to stay away from that. Attempt to complete your exercise essentially a couple of hours before sleep time to give your body time to slow down and unwind.

20 Impacts of not getting sufficient sleep

Not getting sufficient sleep can have a scope of adverse consequences on your physical and psychological wellness. The following are 20 normal impacts of lack of sleep:

1: Fatigue and lack of energy are two of the most common side effects of not getting enough sleep. Your body is unable to properly recharge and repair itself when you don't get enough sleep, which makes you feel tired and sluggish. Concentration, staying focused, and successfully completing tasks can be difficult as a result.

Weakness can likewise influence your actual exhibition, making it harder to practice or participate in actual work. It's possible that you won't have enough energy to finish the things you normally do every day, making it hard to get through the day without getting tired.
Chronic fatigue syndrome, which is characterized by extreme tiredness and exhaustion that does not improve with rest, can also be caused by long-term sleep deprivation. A person's quality of life can be greatly impacted by this debilitating condition.

It is essential to place a high priority on getting enough sleep each night in order to combat fatigue and a lack of energy brought on by sleep deprivation. This might include changing your rest plan, loosening up your sleep time schedule, and making changes to your way of life and climate to advance better rest.

2: Memory and concentration issues are another common side effect of insufficient sleep. At the point when you don't get sufficient rest, it tends to be hard to concentrate and focus on errands, and you might think of yourself as quickly flustered or absent minded. This can be especially challenging when working on projects or studying that require constant focus.

Memory formation and consolidation may also be hindered by sleep deprivation. The brain processes and consolidates the day's memories during sleep; consequently, this process is disrupted when you don't get enough sleep. This can make it hard to remember specifics or information, which can make it harder to learn and remember new information.

Sleep deprivation can have an effect on memory and concentration as well as on cognitive function and decision-making. You might have trouble processing information and making logical connections or making decisions that are rash or risky.

To battle unfortunate focus and memory issues brought about by lack of sleep, focusing on getting sufficient rest every night is significant. To improve your sleep hygiene, you might want to establish a regular sleep schedule, practice relaxation techniques before going to bed, and modify your lifestyle and surroundings. Additionally, regular exercise and a healthy diet can aid in cognitive function and mental clarity, so you might want to think about including them in your routine.

3: Irritability and mood swings are two additional common side effects of not getting enough sleep. Sleep deprivation can cause mood and emotion changes, which can make you more likely to be irritable, tense, and prone to mood swings. Your interpersonal relationships and ability to carry out day-to-day activities may be impacted by this.

Your body produces less serotonin, a neurotransmitter that controls mood and emotions, when you don't get enough sleep. Anxiety, depression, and irritability can result from this. Sleep deprivation can also lead to an increase in the production of stress hormones like cortisol, which can make mood swings even worse.

A lack of sleep for an extended period of time can also raise one's risk of developing mood disorders like anxiety and depression. In fact, research has shown that compared to people who get enough sleep, insomniacs are more likely to develop depression.
It is essential to place a high priority on getting enough sleep each night in order to combat irritability and mood swings brought on by lack of sleep. This might include making a steady rest plan, rehearsing unwinding procedures before sleep time, and making changes to your way of life and climate to advance better rest cleanliness. If you're having emotional difficulties or mood swings, you might want to talk to a mental health professional for help.

4: One more typical impact of not getting sufficient rest is increased pressure and uneasiness. Lack of sleep can

cause changes in the body's pressure reaction, prompting
an expansion in pressure chemicals like cortisol.
Anxiety, nervousness, and tension can result from this,
making it harder to unwind and relax.
A vicious cycle of stress and sleep deprivation can also
be exacerbated by sleep deprivation. While you're
feeling worried, it tends to be challenging to nod off or
stay unconscious, prompting further lack of sleep and an
expansion in pressure chemicals.

Anxiety disorders like panic disorder and generalized
anxiety disorder have also been linked to an increased
risk of chronic sleep deprivation. This might be on the
grounds that absence of rest can prompt changes in mind
science and capability, influencing temperament and
profound guidelines.

It is essential to place a high priority on getting enough
sleep each night in order to combat the increased stress
and anxiety brought on by lack of sleep. This might
include making a reliable rest plan, rehearsing
unwinding procedures before sleep time, and making
changes to your way of life and climate to advance better
rest cleanliness. If you're having trouble managing stress

or anxiety, you might also want to think about speaking
with a mental health professional for help. They might
be able to offer you coping mechanisms and assist you in
making a strategy for dealing with your symptoms.

5: A rise in the likelihood of developing long-term
health issues is yet another common side effect of not
getting enough sleep. Obesity, diabetes, cardiovascular
disease, and impaired immune function have all been
linked to sleep deprivation.

The body's metabolism can be impacted by sleep
deprivation, which can contribute to these health issues.
Your body produces more of the hunger-inducing
hormone ghrelin and less of the appetite-controlling
hormone leptin when you don't get enough sleep. This
may increase appetite and food intake, which may
contribute to obesity and weight gain.

Insulin resistance, a condition in which the body's cells
become less responsive to insulin, a hormone that helps
regulate blood sugar levels, has also been linked to sleep
deprivation. Type 2 diabetes, a chronic condition

characterized by high blood sugar levels, may develop as a result of this.

Sleep deprivation can also alter the cardiovascular system of the body, increasing the likelihood of developing cardiovascular disease and hypertension. Sleep deprivation has also been linked to an increased risk of heart attack and stroke.
Finally, getting too little sleep can make it harder for the body to fight off illnesses and infections. As a result, you may be more likely to catch colds, flu, and other infections.

It is essential to place a high priority on getting enough sleep each night in order to combat the increased risk of chronic health conditions brought on by sleep deprivation. This might include making a reliable rest plan, rehearsing unwinding methods before sleep time, and making changes to your way of life and climate to advance better rest cleanliness. You might also want to talk to a doctor about how likely you are to develop chronic health conditions and make a plan for managing your overall health.

6 : A weakened immune system is another common side effect of not getting enough sleep. Sleep deprivation can make you more likely to get sick because it can affect how well your body can fight off illnesses and infections.

Cytokines are proteins produced by the body while it is asleep that aid in infection prevention and immune system control. At the point when you don't get sufficient rest, the development of cytokines diminishes, making it harder for the body to ward off infections and microscopic organisms.
Sleep deprivation can also lead to an increase in stress hormones like cortisol, which can make the immune system even weaker. A variety of illnesses, including the common cold, the flu, and other infections, have been linked to an increased risk of chronic sleep deprivation.

Prioritizing getting enough sleep each night is essential in order to combat the weakened immune system brought on by sleep deprivation. To improve your sleep hygiene, you might want to establish a regular sleep schedule, practice relaxation techniques before going to bed, and modify your lifestyle and surroundings. You might also think about improving your immune system as a whole by getting regular exercise, eating a healthy diet, and avoiding bad habits like smoking and drinking too much alcohol.

If you do fall ill, it's critical to put rest and recovery first by getting more sleep and taking breaks from work and other activities as needed. This could help make sure that your body has what it needs to fight off illness and get better faster.

7: Impaired cognitive function is another common side effect of not getting enough sleep. The brain's capacity for information processing, memory consolidation, and emotion regulation all depend on adequate sleep. At the point when you don't get sufficient rest, these cycles can be disturbed, prompting a scope of mental impedances.

Impaired memory and concentration are among the most obvious cognitive effects of sleep deprivation. It can be harder to concentrate, remember information, and complete mental-intensive tasks when you don't get enough sleep. This can have an impact not only on how well you perform at work or school but also on everyday activities like driving or making decisions.

Sleep deprivation can also have an effect on mood and emotional regulation, making it harder to control stress and keep your emotions in check. Anxiety, depression, and irritability are all possible outcomes of this.
Also, lack of sleep has been connected to an expanded gamble of mishaps and wounds, especially those that include driving or working large equipment. This is on the grounds that lack of sleep can debilitate response time, judgment, and coordination.

To battle debilitated mental capability brought about by lack of sleep, focusing on getting sufficient rest every night is significant. To improve your sleep hygiene, you might want to establish a regular sleep schedule, practice relaxation techniques before going to bed, and modify your lifestyle and surroundings. You might also want to think about taking breaks throughout the day to unwind your mind and giving priority to activities like exercise and meditation, both of which can improve mood and cognitive function.

Talk to a healthcare provider or mental health professional if, despite getting enough sleep, you continue to struggle with cognitive impairments. They can give you a full evaluation and help you make a plan for how to deal with your symptoms.

8: One more typical impact of not getting sufficient rest is an expanded gamble of mishaps and wounds. Sleep deprivation can slow down reaction time, make it harder to focus on things, and make it harder to work together.

Driving is one area where this is especially concerning. Sleep deprivation has been shown to have the same effect on driving ability as drinking alcohol, raising the risk of road accidents and injuries. Drowsy driving is responsible for an estimated 100,000 accidents and 1,500 deaths each year in the United States alone, according to the National Highway Traffic Safety Administration.

Sleep deprivation can also make it more likely that someone will get hurt at work, especially if the accident involves heavy machinery or dangerous materials. Sleep deprivation can affect judgment and coordination, making it harder to safely operate machinery and react quickly to unforeseen circumstances.

It is essential to place a high priority on getting enough sleep each night in order to combat the increased risk of accidents and injuries brought on by sleep deprivation. To improve your sleep hygiene, you might want to establish a regular sleep schedule, practice relaxation techniques before going to bed, and modify your lifestyle and surroundings.

It's especially important to get enough sleep before driving or operating machinery if you know you'll be doing so. You could also think about taking breaks during long drives or shifts at work to rest your mind and avoid getting tired.
Last but not least, speaking with a healthcare professional may be beneficial if, despite getting enough sleep, you are experiencing persistent fatigue or sleepiness. They can assist you in evaluating any underlying conditions that might be affecting your ability to sleep and offer you strategies for managing fatigue and remaining alert throughout the day.

9: An increased risk of weight gain and obesity is
another common side effect of not getting enough sleep.
When you don't get enough sleep, hormones that control
appetite and metabolism can become out of balance.
Sleep plays a crucial role in this process.
Sleep deprivation has been linked to elevated levels of
the appetite-stimulating hormone ghrelin and decreased
levels of the hunger-satisfying hormone leptin,
according to studies. This can increase food intake and
increase the likelihood of overeating, particularly of
foods high in fat and calories.

Sleep deprivation has also been linked to metabolic
changes that can lead to obesity and weight gain. Insulin
resistance is a condition in which the body has trouble
using insulin to control blood sugar levels and can be
caused by not getting enough sleep. Obesity and type 2
diabetes may be more likely as a result of this.
To battle the expanded gamble of weight gain and
heftiness brought about by lack of sleep, focusing on
getting sufficient rest every night is significant. This
might include making a predictable rest plan, rehearsing
unwinding strategies before sleep time, and making

changes to your way of life and climate to advance better rest cleanliness.

In addition, if you want to maintain a healthy weight, changing your eating and exercise routines might be beneficial. Increasing your level of physical activity, reducing your intake of high-calorie, high-fat foods, and prioritizing a well-balanced diet with plenty of fruits, vegetables, and whole grains are all possible ways to accomplish this.

At long last, in the event that you're battling with tireless weight gain regardless of making lifestyle changes, it could be useful to talk with a medical services supplier or enrolled dietitian. They can assist you in evaluating any underlying conditions that may be affecting your weight and provide you with individual weight management and health-promoting strategies.

10: An increased risk of cardiovascular disease is another common side effect of not getting enough sleep. Blood pressure, inflammation, and blood sugar levels are just a few of the processes that are important for heart health that are regulated by sleep. These processes can

be disrupted if you don't get enough sleep, which can
raise your risk of cardiovascular disease.
Blood pressure can rise when a person doesn't get
enough sleep, especially at night when the body is
usually at rest, according to studies. A major risk factor
for cardiovascular disease, including heart attacks and
strokes, is high blood pressure.

Atherosclerosis is a condition in which plaque builds up
in the arteries and prevents blood flow, and sleep
deprivation has also been linked to an increase in
inflammation in the body. Heart attacks, strokes, and
other cardiovascular events may be more likely as a
result.

Last but not least, lack of sleep has been linked to an
increase in insulin resistance, a condition in which the
body has trouble using insulin to control blood sugar
levels. Insulin resistance is another major risk factor for
cardiovascular disease that can contribute to the
development of type 2 diabetes.
It is essential to place a high priority on getting enough
sleep each night in order to combat the increased risk of
cardiovascular disease brought on by sleep deprivation.

To improve your sleep hygiene, you might want to establish a regular sleep schedule, practice relaxation techniques before going to bed, and modify your lifestyle and surroundings.

A healthy lifestyle that includes regular exercise, a well-balanced diet, and strategies for managing stress is also essential. The risk of cardiovascular disease can be decreased and overall heart health can be improved through these methods.
Talking to a doctor may be beneficial if you struggle with chronic lack of sleep or have a family history of cardiovascular disease. They can help you figure out how likely you are to get cardiovascular disease and give you individual plans to lower your risk and improve your overall health.

11: A higher risk of depression and other mental health issues is another effect of not getting enough sleep. When you don't get enough sleep, the processes that control your mood, emotions, and cognitive function can be disrupted, increasing your risk of developing mental health issues. Sleep plays a crucial role in mood, emotion, and cognitive function regulation.

Sleep deprivation has been linked to an increase in depression symptoms like sadness, hopelessness, and irritability, according to research. Anxiety disorders and other mental health conditions have also been linked to a higher risk of sleep deprivation.

Sleep deprivation can also have an effect on memory, attention, and decision-making, among other cognitive functions. This can make things harder at work or school, as well as make accidents and other safety issues more likely.

Prioritize getting enough sleep each night in order to combat the increased risk of depression and other mental health issues brought on by sleep deprivation. To improve your sleep hygiene, you might want to establish a regular sleep schedule, practice relaxation techniques before going to bed, and modify your lifestyle and surroundings.

Likewise, it's critical to look for treatment for any psychological wellness issues you might be encountering, like despondency or tension. Talking to a mental health professional, taking medication, or participating in therapy or other treatments are all examples of this.

Last but not least, a healthy lifestyle that includes regular exercise, a well-balanced diet, and strategies for managing stress is essential. These systems can assist with decreasing the gamble of psychological well-being issues and advance by and large prosperity.

Talking to a healthcare professional may be beneficial if you struggle with mental health issues or sleep deprivation on a regular basis. They can assist you in evaluating your symptoms and providing you with individualized approaches to managing your mental and sleep health.

12 : Impairment of the immune system: A healthy immune system depends on getting enough sleep, and not getting enough can make it harder for your body to fight off diseases and infections. Cytokines are proteins produced by the immune system during sleep that aid in the fight against stress, infection, and inflammation. These cytokines can be less produced when people don't get enough sleep, which makes it harder for the body to

fight off illnesses and infections. Additionally, insufficient sleep has been linked to an increased risk of the common cold, flu, and other infections, according to studies.

13 : Greater danger of accidents: Lack of sleep can influence mental capability and response time, making it harder to think, decide, and respond rapidly in circumstances that require consideration and concentration. This can expand the gamble of mishaps, including auto collisions, falls, and work environment wounds. As a matter of fact, studies have demonstrated the way that lack of sleep can debilitate driving execution in a manner that is like driving affected by liquor.
It is essential to place a high priority on getting enough sleep each night in order to combat the increased risk of accidents and impaired immune function brought on by sleep deprivation. To improve your sleep hygiene, you might want to establish a regular sleep schedule, practice relaxation techniques before going to bed, and modify your lifestyle and surroundings.

In addition, in order to lower your risk of contracting an infection, it is essential to adhere to good hygiene practices such as regularly washing your hands, covering your mouth when coughing or sneezing, and avoiding close contact with sick people.

Last but not least, it's important to avoid accidents and be aware of the dangers of not getting enough sleep. When you're feeling sleepy, this could mean avoiding activities that require a lot of concentration or physical coordination and taking breaks or naps whenever you need to recharge your mind and body.

14: Not getting enough sleep can also make you more likely to gain weight and become obese. Studies have shown that individuals who don't get sufficient rest consistently are bound to have a higher weight list (BMI) and to be overweight or hefty.

Lack of sleep can lead to weight gain for a number of reasons. One possibility is that hormones like leptin and ghrelin, which control appetite and metabolism, can be affected by lack of sleep. Ghrelin is a hormone that increases appetite and encourages food intake, while leptin is a hormone that tells the brain when you're full and should stop eating. Your body produces more ghrelin and less leptin when you don't get enough sleep, which can make you feel hungry and less satisfied after eating.

Also, lack of sleep can influence your body's capacity to process and utilize insulin, which can prompt insulin opposition and an expanded gamble of creating type 2 diabetes. By making it more difficult for the body to use glucose as a source of energy and by encouraging fat storage, insulin resistance can also contribute to obesity and weight gain.

Prioritize getting enough sleep each night in order to combat the increased risk of obesity and weight gain brought on by sleep deprivation. To improve your sleep hygiene, you might want to establish a regular sleep schedule, avoid alcohol and caffeine before bed, and modify your lifestyle and surroundings.

To support a healthy weight, it's also important to eat well and exercise frequently. This may necessitate regular physical activity, such as walking, jogging, or lifting weights, as well as a well-balanced diet rich in fruits, vegetables, lean protein, and whole grains.

A conversation with a medical professional may be beneficial if you are experiencing persistent sleep deprivation or weight gain. They are able to assist in the evaluation of your symptoms and provide you with individual strategies for managing your weight and sleep.

15: One more impact of not getting sufficient rest is an expanded gamble of psychological wellness issues like sadness and nervousness. Studies have demonstrated the way that lack of sleep can adversely affect state of mind and profound prosperity, prompting side effects of melancholy and tension.

The body's stress response system, which is in charge of regulating the body's response to stress and anxiety, is regulated by sleep. Stress hormones like cortisol, which can disrupt the body's stress response system and contribute to feelings of anxiety and depression, can rise as a result of chronic sleep deprivation.

Sleep deprivation can also have an effect on memory, cognitive function, and decision-making skills, which can have an effect on emotional regulation and raise the risk of having negative emotional states. Sleep deprivation has also been linked to less social

interaction, which can make people feel lonely and
socially isolated, which are both risk factors for
depression and anxiety.
It is essential to place a high priority on getting enough
sleep each night in order to combat the increased risk of
depression and anxiety brought on by lack of sleep. To
improve your sleep hygiene, you might want to establish
a regular sleep schedule, avoid alcohol and caffeine
before bed, and modify your lifestyle and surroundings.

To support mental health and emotional well-being, it's
important to practice self-care activities like exercise,
meditation, or therapy. Talking to a healthcare provider
or mental health professional may be beneficial if you
are experiencing mental health issues or persistent sleep
deprivation. They can assist you in evaluating your
symptoms and providing you with individualized
approaches to managing your mental and sleep health.

16 : One more impact of not getting sufficient rest is an
expanded gamble of mishaps and wounds. Sleep
deprivation can have a negative impact on cognitive
function, reaction time, and decision-making abilities,

making it more challenging to respond appropriately to
hazards and unanticipated circumstances.

People who don't get enough sleep are more likely to be
in car accidents, workplace accidents, and other kinds of
accidents that can hurt them, according to research.
Additionally, falling has been linked to an increased risk,
which is especially dangerous for older adults.

Sleep deprivation not only has a direct effect on safety,
but it can also contribute to long-term health issues like
obesity, diabetes, and cardiovascular disease, which can
make it more likely that a person will become disabled
in the future.

It is essential to place a priority on getting enough sleep
each night in order to reduce the likelihood of accidents
and injuries brought on by lack of sleep. To improve
your sleep hygiene, you might want to establish a regular
sleep schedule, avoid alcohol and caffeine before bed,
and modify your lifestyle and surroundings.
Sleep is especially important if you work in
transportation, construction, or healthcare, which all
place a high value on safety, so you can do your job

safely and effectively. Additionally, employers may have programs and policies in place to encourage employee sleep and workplace safety.

Be aware of the symptoms of sleep deprivation, such as excessive sleepiness, difficulty concentrating, and changes in mood, and take steps to address these symptoms if they occur, in addition to these measures. Talk to a doctor or safety professional if you're worried about your sleep or if you've been in an accident or been hurt because you didn't get enough sleep. They can assist you in evaluating your symptoms and providing you with customized sleep management and injury risk reduction strategies.

17: Getting too little sleep can also make you more likely to get heart disease. Constant lack of sleep has been connected to various gambling factors for cardiovascular illness, including hypertension, diabetes, and weight.

The cardiovascular system of the body, including the function of the heart and blood vessels, is tightly controlled by sleep. Sleep deprivation can interfere with these processes and raise blood pressure, inflammation, and other cardiovascular risk factors.

According to research, people who get seven to eight hours of sleep per night are less likely to develop cardiovascular disease than those who get less than six hours of sleep per night on a regular basis. Additionally, sleep apnea and other related sleep disorders have been linked to an increased risk of cardiovascular disease, particularly in older adults.

It is essential to place a high priority on getting enough sleep each night in order to reduce the risk of cardiovascular disease brought on by sleep deprivation. To improve your sleep hygiene, you might want to establish a regular sleep schedule, avoid alcohol and caffeine before bed, and modify your lifestyle and surroundings.

What's more, it's essential to keep a solid way of life, including eating a decent eating routine, participating in ordinary actual work, and overseeing pressure. All of these factors have the potential to improve cardiovascular health and lower the likelihood of developing chronic disease.

Snoring or excessive daytime sleepiness are signs of a sleep disorder, so it's important to talk to a doctor. They

can assist you in evaluating your symptoms and
providing you with customized sleep management and
cardiovascular disease risk reduction strategies.

18 : A higher risk of mental health issues is another
effect of not getting enough sleep. Chronic lack of sleep
can have a negative impact on mental health because
sleep is essential for mood, emotion, and cognitive
function regulation.

People who consistently get less than seven hours of
sleep per night are more likely to experience depression
and anxiety symptoms, according to studies. Sleep
deprivation can also make it harder to manage symptoms
of mental health conditions that are already present.

Sleep deprivation has also been linked to an increased
risk of bipolar disorder, schizophrenia, and substance
abuse disorders, in addition to depression and anxiety.
Sleep deprivation can also have an effect on cognitive
function, such as memory, attention, and decision-
making, which can have an effect on relationships and
daily life.

Prioritizing getting enough sleep each night is essential to lowering the likelihood of developing mental health issues as a result of sleep deprivation. To improve your sleep hygiene, you might want to establish a regular sleep schedule, avoid alcohol and caffeine before bed, and modify your lifestyle and surroundings.

To support mental health, it's also important to practice stress management and self-care. This might include participating in unwinding procedures like contemplation or yoga, looking for help from loved ones, or working with a psychological wellness expert to foster survival techniques.
It's important to talk to a doctor if you're having symptoms of depression, anxiety, or any other mental health issue. They can assist you in evaluating your symptoms and providing you with customized sleep management and mental health improvement strategies.

19: Getting too little sleep can also make accidents and injuries more likely. Lack of sleep can disable mental capability, response time, and independent direction, which can prompt a more serious gamble of mishaps and wounds both on and off the gig.

Sleep deprivation has been linked to an increased risk of car accidents, workplace accidents, and other kinds of accidents, according to studies. Furthermore, individuals who reliably get under six hours of rest each night are bound to participate in hazardous ways of behaving, like driving affected by medications or liquor.

Sleep deprivation can also be bad for your physical health, making you more likely to have chronic pain and other health problems that make it hard to do things every day and make you more likely to get into accidents and injuries.

To lessen the gamble of mishaps and wounds brought about by lack of sleep, focusing on getting sufficient rest every night is significant. To improve your sleep hygiene, you might want to establish a regular sleep schedule, avoid alcohol and caffeine before bed, and modify your lifestyle and surroundings.
Good sleep habits like avoiding screen time before bed, creating a comfortable sleeping environment, and practicing relaxation techniques like deep breathing or meditation are also important.

It is essential to consult a medical professional if you are exhibiting signs of sleep deprivation, such as excessive daytime sleepiness or difficulty concentrating. They can assist you in evaluating your symptoms and providing you with customized sleep management and injury risk reduction strategies.

20 : A weakened immune system is the final effect of not getting enough sleep. Sleep is very important for keeping the immune system working right, and getting too little sleep can make it harder for the immune system to fight off illnesses and infections.
People who consistently get less than seven hours of sleep per night are more likely to catch colds, flu, and other respiratory infections, according to research. Sleep deprivation can also make people more likely to develop long-term conditions like diabetes, heart disease, and obesity, which can further weaken the immune system and make it more likely to get sick.
It is essential to place a high priority on getting enough sleep each night in order to support the immune system and lower the likelihood of contracting illnesses and infections brought on by lack of sleep. To improve your sleep hygiene, you might want to establish a regular

sleep schedule, avoid alcohol and caffeine before bed, and modify your lifestyle and surroundings.

In order to lessen the likelihood of contracting an infection, it's also critical to adhere to good hygiene practices like hand washing on a regular basis and avoiding close contact with sick people.

It's important to talk to a doctor if you have symptoms of not getting enough sleep or a weaker immune system. They can assist you in evaluating your symptoms and providing you with customized sleep management and immune system support strategies.

Chapter 8

Manage stress

Taking proactive measures to lessen the negative effects of stress on your physical and emotional health is part of stress management. Identifying the things in your life that cause you stress, learning how to cope with stress, and making changes to your lifestyle to reduce stress are all examples of this. Overseeing pressure can assist with diminishing the gamble of creating medical conditions connected with persistent pressure, for example, hypertension, coronary illness, and sadness. You can promote a greater sense of well-being and improve your overall quality of life by managing stress.

We as a whole encounter pressure. It's just part of life. However, excessive stress can harm our kidneys and contribute to poor health by raising blood pressure. We can maintain kidney health and overall health by understanding how stress affects our health and finding ways to manage it.

Anything that can cause you stress is considered to be stress. Stress can be physiological (infection, injury, disease) or psychological (anxiety, disagreement, threats to one's well-being or safety). Living with a constant sickness, like kidney infection, or realizing interestingly that you have an ongoing disease can be a huge wellspring of stress.

Psychological stress is a problem that we face on a daily basis. It can come from positive life events like getting married and having kids, or it can come from more difficult life events like losing a loved one, getting divorced, or having problems with one's finances or personal life.

Your body's response to stress, such as faster breathing and heart rate, a rise in blood pressure, dilated pupils, and tense muscles, is normal and normal. Additionally, your blood sugar and fat levels may rise. The term "fight or flight" refers to the body's response to stress. Stress and Kidney Function can eventually take a toll on your health, despite the fact that it is a natural process that helps us survive immediate dangers. However, excessive or constant stress can cause these reactions.

Our kidney function is one area where stress can have a significant impact on our physical and mental health. The kidneys are a pair of organs in the shape of beans that are in the back of the abdominal cavity. They are responsible for filtering the blood of waste products and excess fluids. They also produce hormones that encourage the production of red blood cells and assist in the regulation of blood pressure.

The body's "fight or flight" response is sparked by stress, which results in the release of hormones like adrenaline and cortisol. By raising the heart rate, blood pressure, and rate of breathing, these hormones prepare the body for a perceived threat. Even though this response is helpful in brief bursts, prolonged high levels of these hormones can be caused by chronic stress, which can be harmful to the kidneys and other organs.

One of the fundamental manners by which stress influences kidney capability is by expanding circulatory strain. By adjusting the body's salt and fluid levels, the kidneys play a crucial role in controlling blood pressure. The kidneys' blood vessels can become damaged when blood pressure rises consistently, reducing their capacity to effectively filter waste products. This could eventually result in chronic kidney disease, which could eventually lead to kidney failure.

Inflammatory cytokines, which can contribute to kidney inflammation and damage, can also be produced by the body in response to stress. Autoimmune diseases like lupus and rheumatoid arthritis, which can also affect kidney function, have been linked to chronic stress.

In addition to having a direct impact on kidney function, stress can also make people engage in unhealthy behaviors like smoking, drinking alcohol, and eating too much, which can make the risk of kidney disease even higher.

Stress management is essential for maintaining kidney health. This could mean doing things like yoga, deep breathing, meditation, or other forms of relaxation, exercising frequently, getting enough sleep, or eating a healthy diet. It's likewise vital to look for clinical consideration on the off chance that you have hypertension or different side effects of kidney sickness, as early intercession can assist with forestalling further harm.

Ways To Decrease Your Stress

It is extremely challenging, if not impossible, to completely eliminate stress or to never experience any physical responses to stress. However, there are things you can do to help control your body's response to stress

and manage stress. A basic ways of decreasing your
stress include:

1.Reduce your intake of salt, caffeine, and sugar
(especially if you have diabetes)

2. fats (especially if you are at risk for heart and blood
vessel disease) for a healthier diet.

3. Schedule time to unwind using relaxation techniques
(yoga, meditation, etc.)

4. Talk to a friend, a loved one, a spiritual leader, or a
medical professional.

5.Vacation Regular exercise and more physical
activity.

Chapter 9

Monitor your kidney health

Your kidneys are essential to your body because they control the fluid balance and remove waste products from the blood. It is essential for your overall health and well-being to maintain kidney health. It is essential to see a doctor if you have any symptoms related to kidney function or are at risk for kidney disease.

It is critical to keep track of how quickly or slowly your kidney disease progresses. The proportion of your kidneys that are still functioning is known as your kidney function. By monitoring your serum creatinine, which is a waste product found in your blood and can be checked with a simple blood test, you and your doctor will be able to ascertain this. In order to begin the best therapy, it is essential to meet with your healthcare team on a regular basis and to have tests performed to detect issues and complications early.

Kidney failure can be treated in a variety of ways. Dialysis, which can remove waste in close proximity to a functioning kidney, is one of these treatments and medications that can slow down kidney disease.

when to see a doctor

1.Changes in urine : can allude to any adjustment in the recurrence, variety, smell, volume, or stream of pee. These changes could be signs of a number of different underlying medical conditions, and they could be short-term or ongoing. Urinary changes include the following:

2.Frequency increases: This might be an indication of a urinary plot contamination, prostate issues, diabetes, or pregnancy.

3.Reduction in frequency: This might show lack of hydration or an impediment in the urinary plot.

4.Urinary discomfort: This could be a sign of kidney stones, a sexually transmitted infection, or an infection of the urinary tract.

5.Urine with blood: This might demonstrate a urinary parcel disease, kidney stones, or bladder malignant growth.

6.Shady or putrid urine: This could be a sign of an infection in the urinary tract.

7.Having trouble urinating: An enlarged prostate or a urinary tract obstruction could be the cause of this.

8.Incontinence urinating: This is the involuntary leakage of urine and can be brought on by medications, nerve damage, weak pelvic muscles, or both.
If you notice any changes in your urination, you should talk to a doctor right away because some conditions might need treatment right away.

9. Swelling : A medical condition characterized by an abnormal accumulation of fluid in the body's tissues is known as swelling, edema, or inflammation. This can happen in different pieces of the body, including the feet, lower legs, legs, hands, arms, and face. Injury, infection, allergic reactions, hormonal imbalances, certain

medications, and underlying medical conditions are all
potential causes of swelling.

A variety of symptoms, including pain, tenderness,
warmth, redness, stiffness, and limited range of motion,
can be brought on by swelling. Additionally, the affected
area's skin may appear shiny, stretched, or discolored in
some instances. Swelling can be acute, which means it
happens suddenly and lasts a short time, or chronic,
which means it lasts for a longer time.

To treat enlarging, the basic reason should be recognized
and tended to. Treatment might include the utilization of
meds, for example, diuretics to decrease liquid
development, mitigating medications to diminish
aggravation, or antimicrobials to treat contaminations.
Compression garments, elevating the affected area, or
applying ice packs to alleviate pain and swelling are
other options.

Swelling can result in more serious problems like
decreased blood flow, impaired organ function, and
tissue damage if it is not treated. If swelling is severe or

comes with other symptoms like fever or trouble
breathing, it's important to see a doctor.

A feeling of physical or mental exhaustion known as
fatigue is frequently referred to as a lack of energy or
drive to complete tasks. It can be brought on by a
number of things, like working out too much, not getting
enough sleep, eating poorly, being stressed, being sick,
or having side effects from medications.

A decrease in physical strength, endurance, and overall
energy levels are typically signs of physical fatigue. It
may be challenging to engage in physical activities like
exercise or manual labor as a result of this. In addition to
physical fatigue, muscle weakness, joint pain, and
coordination problems may occur.

However, cognitive abilities like memory, attention, and
decision-making are impacted by mental exhaustion.
Reduced mental clarity, forgetfulness, and difficulty
concentrating are all possible outcomes of this.
Individuals encountering mental exhaustion may

likewise feel peevish or experience issues managing
their feelings.

A medical condition known as chronic fatigue syndrome
(CFS) is characterized by severe and unrelenting fatigue
that does not respond to rest. It can likewise cause
different side effects, for example, muscle agony,
migraines, and weakened mental capability. Although
the precise cause of CFS is unknown, it is believed to be
linked to a combination of psychological, environmental,
and genetic factors.

A person's ability to work, participate in social activities,
and carry out day-to-day activities can all be negatively
impacted by fatigue, which can have a significant impact
on their quality of life. In order to manage symptoms
and improve overall health and well-being, it is essential
to address the underlying causes of fatigue and, if
necessary, seek medical attention.

Conclusion

Your overall health and well-being depend on having
healthy kidneys. This book shows you how to keep your

kidneys healthy and avoid developing kidney disease
with easy-to-follow steps. The book is written well and
easy to understand, making it a useful resource for
kidney health improvement. You can take control of
your health and ensure that your kidneys are functioning
at their best if you follow the advice in this book.

www.ingramcontent.com/pod-product-compliance
Lightning Source LLC
Chambersburg PA
CBHW061634250726
48659CB00004B/1213